Poisoning - New Insights

Edited by Suna Sabuncuoğlu

Published in London, United Kingdom

Poisoning - New Insights
http://dx.doi.org/10.5772/intechopen.1006250
Edited by Suna Sabuncuoğlu

Contributors
Ehab Aki, Hermann Fromme, Katrin Romanek, Manfred Wildner, Martin Socher, Mohamed Elgassim,
Mohammed Abdurabu, Mutwakil Elbidairi, Sumitra Debnath, Suna Sabuncuoğlu, Thomas Zilker

Notice

Statements and opinions expressed in the chapters are these of the individual contributors and not
necessarily those of the editors or publisher. No responsibility is accepted for the accuracy of
information contained in the published chapters. The publisher assumes no responsibility for any
damage or injury to persons or property arising out of the use of any materials, instructions, methods
or ideas contained in the book.

First published in London, United Kingdom, 2025 by IntechOpen
IntechOpen is the global imprint of INTECHOPEN LIMITED, registered in England and Wales,
registration number: 11086078, 167-169 Great Portland Street, London, W1W 5PF, United Kingdom

For EU product safety concerns: IN TECH d.o.o., Prolaz Marije Krucifikse Kozulić 3, 51000 Rijeka,
Croatia, info@intechopen.com or visit our website at intechopen.com.

British Library Cataloguing-in-Publication Data
A catalogue record for this book is available from the British Library

Poisoning - New Insights
Edited by Suna Sabuncuoğlu
p. cm.
Print ISBN 978-1-83634-860-3
Online ISBN 978-1-83634-859-7
eBook (PDF) ISBN 978-1-83634-861-0

If disposing of this product, please recycle the paper responsibly.

IntechOpen

intechopen.com

Built by scientists, for scientists

Meet the editor

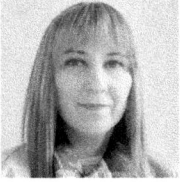

Suna Sabuncuoğlu graduated from Hacettepe University, Faculty of Pharmacy, in 2001. She began working as a research assistant in the Department of Pharmaceutical Toxicology at the same faculty in 2002. She completed her Master's degree in 2005 and her Ph.D. in 2010. During her doctoral studies, she spent one year at the International Agency for Research on Cancer (IARC) in Lyon, France, as an Erasmus student. Following her Ph.D., she conducted postdoctoral research at KU Leuven (Catholic University of Leuven), Belgium. In 2013, she was appointed as a lecturer, and in 2014, she received the title of Associate Professor. In 2022, she was promoted to the rank of Professor. She currently continues her academic work as a faculty member in the Department of Pharmaceutical Toxicology at Hacettepe University, Faculty of Pharmacy. In addition to her undergraduate and graduate teaching and research activities, she has held various administrative roles. Since 2014, she has served as a board member of the Hacettepe University Substance and Alcohol Addiction Research and Application Center. She also serves as the Vice Chair of the Department of Professional Pharmaceutical Sciences and as the Assistant Erasmus Coordinator of the Faculty of Pharmacy.

Contents

Preface

Poisoning, as both a scientific concept and a societal challenge, remains one of the most persistently relevant topics in medicine and public health. Modern toxicology shows a much more complicated and multidimensional reality, even though the paradigm of poisoning has historically conjured ideas of acute, high-dose exposures or deliberate acts. Toxic exposures are no longer limited to crises; they are now a part of our surroundings, goods, technologies, and even medical procedures.

This book emerges from a recognition that toxicology is no longer limited to the identification and treatment of overt poisoning events, but must now contend with subtle, chronic, and often invisible exposures that shape long-term health outcomes across populations. It reflects a commitment to bridging classical toxicological principles with modern scientific advances, incorporating molecular biology, systems-level diagnostics, and real-time risk assessment tools into a broader framework of understanding.

This volume is intended for clinicians, researchers, public health professionals, and policy-makers who seek both foundational insights and forward-looking perspectives. Our goal is to provide a scientific and conceptual roadmap that informs effective toxicological decision-making in an era marked by complexity, uncertainty, and rapid change.

We extend our gratitude to the many contributors and reviewers whose expertise and critical insights shaped the content of this work. We hope that this book not only informs but also inspires continued inquiry and collaboration across the diverse domains that toxicology now touches.

Dr. Suna Sabuncuoğlu
Professor,
Faculty of Pharmacy,
Department of Toxicology,
Hacettepe University,
Ankara, Turkey

Chapter 1

Introductory Chapter: Contemporary Perspectives on Poisoning and Toxicological Challenges

Suna Sabuncuoğlu

1. Introduction

Poisoning is an enduring and evolving public health threat, affecting populations across all demographics, geographies, and levels of industrial development. While historically associated with intentional harm or accidental exposure, the modern landscape of poisoning is far more diverse and complex. Advances in pharmaceuticals, the proliferation of synthetic chemicals, increasing environmental pollution, and even geopolitical instability have all contributed to new patterns of toxic exposure. Poisoning today may stem from medication misuse, occupational accidents, environmental contaminants, or chemical agents used in acts of terrorism. As a result, healthcare professionals must be equipped with updated and multidisciplinary tools to diagnose, manage, and prevent poisoning under highly variable circumstances [1, 2].

The increasing complexity of poisoning events has placed toxicology at the intersection of multiple disciplines, including emergency medicine, pharmacology, critical care, forensic medicine, and public health. Contemporary toxicology is no longer confined to academic research or poison control centers; it is a critical component of frontline medical care, particularly in emergency departments where clinicians must make rapid, often life-saving decisions based on incomplete information. This has necessitated the development of structured algorithms, early warning systems, and evidence-based antidotal therapies that can be applied in a timely and effective manner [1–3].

Poisoning remains a leading cause of preventable injury and death in many parts of the world. The World Health Organization (WHO) and numerous national health agencies have identified acute poisoning as a major contributor to the global burden of disease, especially in low- and middle-income countries where regulatory controls and medical infrastructure may be limited. In high-income settings, the widespread availability of over-the-counter medications, recreational drugs, and household chemicals presents a different, but equally concerning, set of risks. Furthermore, emerging threats such as synthetic opioids, industrial accidents, and toxic adulterants in illicit substances have redefined the boundaries of traditional toxicology [4–6].

Within this complex context, there is a critical need for comprehensive resources that synthesize current knowledge and present practical, clinically relevant approaches to poisoning. This includes a deeper understanding of toxicokinetics and toxicodynamics, mechanisms of organ-specific toxicity, and antidote pharmacology, as well as non-pharmacological interventions such as extracorporeal removal techniques. In addition, prevention strategies—ranging from public education to regulatory reforms—remain a cornerstone in the fight against poisoning, particularly in pediatric populations and vulnerable occupational groups [1–3].

2. Toxicological advances, diagnostic trends, and global preparedness

Modern toxicology has advanced considerably, not only in terms of scientific understanding but also in diagnostic capability and response preparedness. Laboratory methods such as high-performance liquid chromatography (HPLC), gas chromatography-mass spectrometry (GC-MS), and immunoassays now allow for precise and timely identification of toxic agents [1, 2]. Point-of-care testing, biomonitoring, and digital toxicology databases have empowered clinicians to make more informed decisions at the bedside. Yet, despite technological progress, clinical suspicion, patient history, and physical examination remain essential tools—especially in resource-limited settings [2].

At the heart of toxicological emergencies lies the concept of risk stratification. Patients exposed to toxins present with a broad spectrum of symptoms, ranging from asymptomatic states to life-threatening multiorgan failure. This necessitates a nuanced understanding of dose-response relationships, latency periods, and metabolic pathways. For instance, hepatotoxic drugs such as paracetamol (acetaminophen) may show delayed clinical manifestations [7], while agents like organophosphates may act within minutes. Understanding these distinctions is vital for prioritizing interventions and anticipating complications.

Another critical component of toxicological management is the use of antidotes. While many poisons lack specific antidotes, several key agents—such as N-acetylcysteine, atropine, naloxone, and chelating agents—remain cornerstones of modern toxicology [1, 2]. The rational use of these substances requires familiarity with their pharmacological mechanisms, dosing schedules, contraindications, and potential interactions. At the same time, supportive care—including airway protection, hemodynamic stabilization, and renal support—must not be neglected, as it often determines outcomes regardless of antidote availability.

Global preparedness for toxicological threats has also become increasingly important, particularly in light of recent chemical disasters and deliberate exposures. Events such as the 1995 Tokyo subway sarin attack [4] or widespread methanol poisonings from counterfeit alcohol have underscored the need for coordinated, multidisciplinary response systems. National and regional poison control centers, emergency protocols, and chemical threat registries form the backbone of such preparedness efforts [6]. International cooperation, data sharing, and training programs have enhanced the collective ability to detect and manage toxic exposures on a population scale [5].

Moreover, environmental and occupational toxicology have garnered renewed attention. Airborne pollutants, heavy metals, pesticide residues, and industrial solvents continue to pose significant long-term health risks. Chronic exposure to low levels of toxins is now recognized as a contributor to diseases such as cancer, neurodegenerative disorders, and endocrine dysfunction [3]. This has led to an expanded role for toxicologists in environmental policy-making, occupational safety, and public health surveillance.

Finally, toxicology must address the psychological and social dimensions of poisoning. Intentional self-poisoning and substance misuse require sensitive, multidisciplinary interventions that combine medical, psychiatric, and social support. Education campaigns, mental health integration, and harm reduction programs have emerged as vital tools in reducing the human cost of these exposures.

In sum, toxicology in the twenty-first century is a dynamic, multifaceted discipline that demands ongoing education, interdisciplinary collaboration, and a patient-centered approach. This book seeks to provide healthcare professionals, researchers, and policymakers with the conceptual frameworks and practical tools necessary to navigate the challenges of modern poisoning. By combining current scientific evidence with clinical expertise, it offers a contemporary perspective on one of medicine's oldest but most persistently relevant problems.

Author details

Suna Sabuncuoğlu
Department of Toxicology, Faculty of Pharmacy, Hacettepe University, Ankara, Türkiye

*Address all correspondence to: sunaatasayar@gmail.com

IntechOpen

References

[1] Brent J, Wallace KL, Burkhart KK, Phillips SD, Donovan JW. Critical Care Toxicology: Diagnosis and Management of the Critically Poisoned Patient. 2nd ed. Gewerbestrass, Switzerland: Springer; 2017. DOI: 10.1007/978-3-319-17900-1

[2] Goldfrank LR, Flomenbaum NE, Lewin NA, Howland MA, Hoffman RS, Nelson LS. Goldfrank's Toxicologic Emergencies. 11th ed. New York: McGraw-Hill Education; 2019

[3] Karlson-Stiber C, Persson H. Cytotoxic fungi—An overview. Toxicon. 2003;**42**(4):339-349. DOI: 10.1016/S0041-0101(03)00155-0

[4] Okumura T, Takasu N, Ishimatsu S, et al. Report on 640 victims of the Tokyo subway sarin attack. Annals of Emergency Medicine. 1996;**28**(2):129-135. DOI: 10.1016/S0196-0644(96)70052-5

[5] Watson JC, Rudge JW. Health systems' "surge capacity": State of the art and priorities for future research. The Milbank Quarterly. 2021;**99**(1):146-175. DOI: 10.1111/1468-0009.12458

[6] Kostic MA, Dart RC, Erdman AR. American association of poison control centers' national poison data system (NPDS): 38th annual report. Clinical Toxicology (Philadelphia, PA.). 2021;**59**(12):1282-1472. DOI: 10.1080/15563650.2021.2004155

[7] Lee WM. Acetaminophen (APAP) hepatotoxicity—Isn't it time for APAP to go away? Journal of Hepatology. 2017;**67**(6):1324-1331. DOI: 10.1016/j.jhep.2017.07.005

Chapter 2

Toxicology in Emergency Medicine

Ehab Aki, Mohammed Abdurabu and Mohamed Elgassim

Abstract

Toxicology is a critical component of emergency medicine, requiring rapid assessment and management to prevent morbidity and mortality. This chapter provides a structured approach to poisoned patients, beginning with initial stabilization using airway, breathing, and circulation (ABCs) and a focused history, including the AMPLE mnemonic (Allergies, Medications, Past medical history, Last meal, Events leading to presentation). A key focus is on toxidromes—distinctive clinical syndromes that offer diagnostic clues for poisoning—including cholinergic, anticholinergic, opioid, sympathomimetic, and serotonin syndromes, along with their characteristic signs and treatment strategies. The discussion then shifts to common toxic substances encountered in the emergency department, such as pharmaceuticals (acetaminophen, salicylates, and opioids), illicit drugs (cocaine and amphetamines), environmental toxins (carbon monoxide, pesticides, and heavy metals), and household poisons (ethylene glycol and methanol). For each, toxicokinetic, clinical presentation, diagnostic evaluation, and evidence-based management—including antidotes and supportive care—are addressed. Additionally, the chapter explores decontamination strategies (activated charcoal and whole bowel irrigation), enhanced elimination techniques (hemodialysis and urinary alkalinization), and risk assessment tools to guide disposition decisions. Special considerations for pediatric and geriatric populations, who may present with unique toxicologic challenges, are also discussed. By integrating a systematic clinical approach with key toxicology principles, this chapter equips emergency physicians with the knowledge necessary to recognize, diagnose, and effectively manage toxicologic emergencies, ultimately improving patient outcomes.

Keywords: toxicology, emergency medicine, poisoning, toxidromes, overdose, decontamination, antidotes, toxicokinetic, supportive care, critical care toxicology

1. Introduction

Poisoning is a significant global public health issue. According to data from the World Health Organization in 2012, nearly 190,000 people died from poisoning worldwide, and in 2008, the number of deaths from poisoning surpassed those from motor vehicle accidents. Additionally, the poisoning death rate nearly tripled globally. There has also been an increase in the number of patients presenting to emergency departments due to both intentional and accidental overdoses. These statistics highlight the importance of Toxicology in emergency medicine [1, 2].

IntechOpen

The management of intoxicated patients requires a specific approach due to the complexities involved in diagnosing and treating overdoses. This chapter focuses on the general strategies for handling intoxicated patients, with an emphasis on initial management. It also explores how a patient's history and physical exams can help doctors identify the drugs involved and provides an overview of the mechanisms of action, physical signs, and treatments for the most common toxic substances, including those associated with high mortality and morbidity rates.

2. A general approach to toxicological cases in emergency medicine

The management of poisoned patients in the emergency department involves resuscitation, obtaining a history, conducting a physical examination, and implementing appropriate treatment strategies.

2.1 Resuscitation

The primary considerations for a poisoned patient arriving at the emergency department include securing the airway, ensuring adequate respiration and maintaining circulatory stability. Mechanical ventilation and intubation may be necessary if ventilation is inadequate, intubation with mechanical ventilation may be necessary. Hypotension should be initially treated with an IV fluid bolus (10–20 mL/kg). If the hypotension does not respond to fluids, administering a specific antidote may be necessary. In cases of suspected opioid overdose (e.g., low Glasgow Coma Scale (GCS), respiratory depression, and pinpoint pupils), naloxone (0.1–2.0 mg IV) should be administered. Additionally, blood sugar should be checked, and hypoglycaemia should be treated with a 50% dextrose solution (50 mL) [3].

2.2 History

History is crucial and should be gathered from the patient whenever possible. If the patient is comatose or unable to provide information, collateral details can be obtained from family members, friends, or medical records. This should include any history of psychiatric disorders, previous suicide attempts, drug abuse, or ongoing medication use. The history should also cover factors such as the time and route of exposure, the amount of substance involved, whether the exposure was intentional or accidental, and the availability of drugs at home. Additionally, it is important to check for signs like missing tablets, empty pill bottles, or other relevant materials found near the patient, as well as whether any family members have chronic conditions such as hypertension or diabetes [4].

2.3 Physical examination

A physical examination of a poisoned patient is crucial in identifying the substance involved and any associated toxidromes. The exam should begin with assessing the patient's general appearance and mental status, noting any signs of confusion or agitation. The skin should be checked for cyanosis, flushing, or signs of intravenous drug use, such as track marks. Eye examination is important to assess pupil size, reactivity, and the presence of symptoms like excessive tearing or involuntary eye movements (nystagmus). The presence of any unusual odors, such as garlic, bitter almonds, glue, or alcohol, can offer clues about specific toxins. The oropharynx should be checked for signs of hypersalivation or dryness, while the chest examination includes listening for breath sounds, assessing for bronchorrhea, and wheezing, and assessing heart rate and rhythm. Abdominal examination should include bowel sounds, tenderness, or rigidity, while extremities should be checked for tremors or muscle fasciculations. Finally, inspecting the patient's clothing for any medications or illegal drugs may provide further insight into the cause of poisoning. This thorough examination is key to guiding diagnosis and treatment [3].

2.4 Toxidromes

Mofenson and Greensher introduced the term "toxidrome" in 1970. Toxidromes refer to a set of abnormal physical findings and vital signs that typically occur in response to a particular class of drugs or substances. The most common toxidromes include cholinergic, anticholinergic, sympathomimetic, opioid, and serotonin syndrome [4, 5].

2.4.1 Cholinergic

Individuals with cholinergic toxidrome usually present with "wet" symptoms, which can be easily recalled using the mnemonics "SLUDGE + 3 Killer B's" or "DUMBELLS." These mnemonics summarize the common clinical signs, with "SLUDGE" representing salivation, lacrimation (tearing), urination, defecation, gastrointestinal cramping, and emesis (vomiting), along with the "Killer B's" which include bronchorrhea (excessive mucus), bradycardia (slow heart rate), and bronchospasm (narrowing of the airways). The "DUMBELLS" mnemonic stands for diarrhea, urination, miosis (small pupils), bradycardia, emesis, lacrimation, lethargy, and salivation. The most common causes of cholinergic toxidrome are organophosphate pesticides, carbamates, certain mushrooms, and sarin (a chemical warfare agent) [4].

2.4.2 Anticholinergics

Anticholinergic toxidrome presents with "dry" symptoms, including delirium, tachycardia, dry and flushed skin, dilated pupils, clonus, elevated body temperature, reduced bowel sounds, and urinary retention. A helpful mnemonic to remember these signs is: "Hot as a Hare, Mad as a Hatter, Red as a Beet, Dry as a Bone, Blind as a Bat." The most frequent causes of anticholinergic toxidrome are antihistamines, antiparkinsonian drugs, muscle relaxants, antipsychotics, antidepressants, amantadine, scopolamine, atropine, and certain plants, such as Jimson weed [4].

2.4.3 Sympathomimetics

This toxidrome is characterized by psychomotor agitation, CNS stimulation, elevated blood pressure, fast heartbeat, dilated pupils, increased body temperature, sweating, and, in severe cases, seizures. The most common causes of these symptoms are cocaine and amphetamines [4].

2.4.4 Opioids

The most typical clinical manifestations of opioid toxidrome are bradycardia, hypotension, hypothermia, coma, respiratory depression, and pinpoint pupils (meiosis). An overdose of propoxyphene may result in seizures. But tiny pupils are not always seen; sometimes, like when meperidine and propoxyphene are poisonous, the pupils could seem normal in size [4].

2.4.5 Serotonin syndrome

Patients with serotonin syndrome typically present with altered mental status, high blood pressure, and a rapid heart rate. They may also experience myoclonus, hyperreflexia, hyperthermia, and increased muscle rigidity. The most common causes are interactions or overdoses involving SSRIs [4].

2.5 Decontaminations

Decontaminating a poisoned patient involves both removing the toxin from the patient and preventing further exposure. This can be done through external methods, like washing the patient, or internal methods, such as gastrointestinal decontamination or enhancing toxin elimination.

2.5.1 Gross decontamination

The patient must be fully undressed and given a thorough wash with lots of water. The decontamination process needs to be carried out in a confined space with all garments taken off. Usually, gross decontamination is applied to exposure to chemicals, biological agents, or radiation.

2.5.2 Gastrointestinal decontamination

The gastrointestinal tract can be decontaminated using a variety of techniques, such as gastric lavage and emesis (induced vomiting). Historically, gastric lavage was widespread and ipecac syrup was used to induce vomiting. But these are now rarely recommended due to the lack of supporting evidence and potential risks. These methods may reduce toxin absorption but can also increase complications. Inducing vomiting and gastric lavage might be considered for conscious, alert patients who have ingested a toxic substance within an hour. However, they are contraindicated in cases where the patient has an unprotected airway, ingested corrosive substances or hydrocarbons, or is in an unstable condition, such as being hypotensive or having seizures [6].

2.5.3 Activated charcoal

Activated charcoal is made by superheating carbon materials to increase its surface area. It works by preventing the absorption of toxins in the stomach and intestines but is ineffective against metals, alcohols, corrosives, and lithium. If administered within an hour of intake, the greatest outcomes are obtained. Lack of intestinal motility, gastrointestinal perforation, consumption of caustic substances, and an unprotected airway are among the contraindications (however if the patient is intubated, it can be given via a nasogastric tube). Potential complications from using activated charcoal include aspiration, which can lead to pneumonitis, ARDS, and issues like small bowel obstruction [7].

2.5.4 Whole-bowel irrigation

Whole-bowel irrigation is a process that cleanses the entire gastrointestinal tract to reduce toxin absorption. This is done using a polyethylene glycol solution. It is indicated for substances with slow absorption, such as sustained-release medications, toxins poorly absorbed by activated charcoal (e.g., metals, lithium), and in body packers. Some side effects include vomiting, bloating, and rectal irritation. It is contraindicated in cases where there are absent bowel sounds or a perforation [8].

2.5.5 Enhanced elimination

By speeding up the body's disposal of toxins, enhanced elimination helps lessen the intensity and length of poisoning symptoms. While not routinely used, it is considered in cases of severe toxicity, when there's poor response to supportive care or antidotes, or when the body's natural elimination processes are slow. Methods for enhanced elimination include multiple-dose activated charcoal (MDAC), which is helpful in cases such as carbamazepine, phenobarbital, and disopyramide toxicity. Urinary alkalinization is effective for poisoning with salicylates or phenobarbital. Additionally, extracorporeal methods like hemodialysis, hemofiltration, plasmapheresis, and exchange transfusion can be used for substances such as lithium, carbamazepine, theophylline, salicylates, and toxic alcohols like ethylene glycol and methanol [4].

2.6 Antidotes

A drug known as the antidote can stop further poisoning from some toxins. The table below shows the most common antidote used in the emergency department (see **Table 1**) [4].

Toxin	Antidote
Acetaminophen	• N-Acetylcysteine 150 mg/kg dextrose IV over 15–60 min then 50 mg/kg NAC IV over 4 hrs. Then 100 mg /kg NAC IV over 16 hrs.
Cholinergic (organophosphates, carbamates)	• Atropine 1-2 mg every 2–3 mins, until there is drying of secretions • Pralidoxime (2-PAM) 70 mg/kg IV then infusion at 500 mg/hour
Anticholinesterases	• Physostigmine 0.5–1 mg IV as a slow push over 5 minutes and repeat every 10 min
Benzodiazepines	• Flumazenil 0.2 Mg repeated max dose 2 mg
β-Blockers	• Glucagon 3–10 mg
Calcium channel blockers	• Calcium gluconate 10% 10–30 mL IV
Cyanide	• Vitamin B12 (Hydroxocobalamin) 70 ml/kg IV. • Amyl nitrite • Sodium thiosulfate • Sodium nitrite (3% solution)
Digoxin	• Digoxin Fab 5–10 vials

Toxin	Antidote
Isoniazid	• Pyridoxine (vitamin B6) 70 mg/kg IV (maximum 5 gm).
Methanol, ethylene glycol	• Ethanol: Loading 8 ml/kg of 10% ethanol then 1–2 ml/kg/hour of 10% ethanol
	• Fomepizole: Loading: 15 mg/kg in 100 ml IV over 30 minutes then maintenance:10 mg/kg IV over 30 minutes every 12 hours for 48 hr.
Narcotics	• Naloxone 0.1–0.4 mg, may repeated
Tricyclic antidepressants	• Sodium bicarbonate: 1–2 mEq/kg IV bolus followed by 2 mEq/kg per h IV infusion
Iron	• Desferrioxamine IV infusion dose of 15 mg/kg/hour
Methemoglobinemia	• Methylene Blue 1–2 mg/kg (0.1–0.2 ml/kg of 1% solution) IV slowly over 5 minutes. In case of G6PD, Vitamin C (Ascorbic Acid) 300–1000 mg/day orally in divided doses.
local anesthesia	• Intravenous lipid emulsion 1–1.5 ml/kg 20% IV bolus over 1 minute and Repeat bolus at 3–5 minutes Then infuse 0.25 ml/kg/minute

Table 1
The most common antidotes in the emergency department [4].

3. Common toxic substances encountered in the emergency department

3.1 Acetaminophen poisoning

Since its clinical introduction in 1950, acetaminophen has become one of the most widely used over-the-counter medications for analgesia and antipyresis. However, in the US, it is also the main cause of acute liver failure [9, 10].

3.1.1 Mechanism of action

Acetaminophen is processed in the liver, where it is converted into nontoxic metabolites through glucuronidation (40–67%) and sulfation (20–46%). A hazardous byproduct known as NAPQI is only little formed at regular dosages, which is safely detoxified by conjugation with glutathione (GSH). Glutathione is an important molecule that helps neutralize harmful substances, like NAPQI, through a reaction that requires NADPH. In the case of an overdose, however, the liver's usual processes are overwhelmed, and the pathways that normally handle acetaminophen are saturated. As a result, glutathione is depleted, and NAPQI builds up, causing it to bind to cellular proteins and ultimately leading to liver cell damage and death [11].

3.1.2 Clinical features

In the early stages of acetaminophen toxicity, symptoms are often nonspecific or may not appear at all. The condition progresses through four stages: In *Stage I* (the first 24 hours), patients may experience nausea, vomiting, fatigue, loss of appetite, or be asymptomatic, with blood tests revealing hypokalaemia and metabolic acidosis. In *Stage II* (Days 2–3), symptoms worsen, with nausea, vomiting, right upper abdominal pain, and significant liver damage indicated by elevated liver enzymes (AST and

ALT). *Stage III* (Days 3–4) is the peak of liver damage, where patients may develop coma, encephalopathy, coagulopathy, kidney failure, jaundice, ARDS, sepsis, and cerebral edema. Finally, in *Stage IV* (Days 7–8), patients either begin to recover or progress to multi-organ failure and potential death [12, 13].

3.1.3 Treatment

After stabilizing the patient's airway, breathing, and circulation, the next step is to consider gastrointestinal decontamination, typically with activated charcoal. The primary treatment for acetaminophen overdose is *N-acetylcysteine (NAC)*. NAC helps replenish glutathione levels and can directly neutralize NAPQI, the toxic metabolite of acetaminophen. If administered within 8 hours of ingestion, NAC is highly effective at preventing liver damage. Although NAC is less effective after 8 hours, it still provides benefits, even in severe cases of liver failure. NAC should only be given to patients at risk of liver damage. The *Rumack-Matthew nomogram* is used to assess the risk of liver toxicity based on the acetaminophen level and the time since ingestion, typically within 24 hours. When the nomogram is not applicable—such as when the time of ingestion is unknown or when more than 24 hours have passed—NAC should be administered right away. If liver enzymes (AST, ALT) return to normal and acetaminophen levels are undetectable, NAC treatment can be stopped. Otherwise, NAC should continue.

It is advised to take 140 mg/kg orally first, then 70 mg/kg every 4 hours for 17 doses, or 150 mg/kg intravenously as a loading dose, followed by 50 mg/kg over 4 hours and 100 mg/kg over 16 hours (**Figure 1**) [14–16].

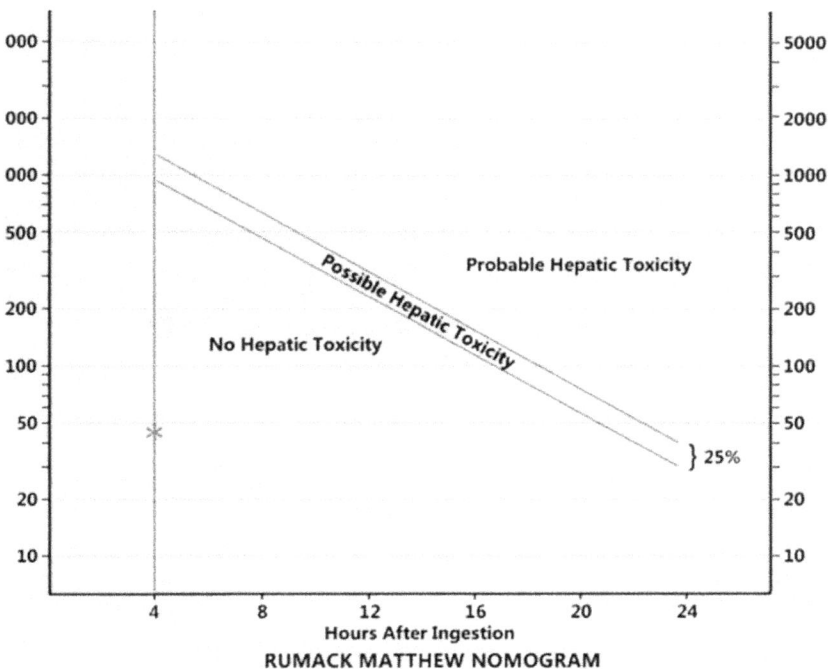

Figure 1
Rumack-Matthew nomogram [14–16].

3.2 Cyclic antidepressants (CA) poisoning

Cyclic antidepressants were once commonly prescribed for depression, but their use has significantly decreased due to the availability of safer alternatives. In fact, in 2013, cyclic antidepressants were the most frequent type of antidepressant involved in overdose-related deaths [17, 18].

3.2.1 Mechanism of action

Cyclic antidepressants (CA) have several pharmacological effects. One of their key actions is their *antihistamine effects*, where they block postsynaptic histamine receptors, leading to sedation, a reduced level of consciousness, and potentially coma. They also have *antimuscarinic effects*, which can be divided into central and peripheral effects. In the central nervous system, blocking acetylcholine receptors can result in agitation, delirium, confusion, hallucinations, slurred speech, ataxia, and even coma. On the peripheral level, blocking acetylcholine receptors causes symptoms such as dilated pupils, tachycardia, hyperthermia, high blood pressure, dry skin, ileus, urinary retention, increased muscle tone, and tremors. Additionally, cyclic antidepressants *inhibit α-adrenergic receptors*, which can lead to sedation, orthostatic hypotension, tachycardia, and pupillary constriction, although the antimuscarinic effects typically counteract the pupillary dilation. The *inhibition of amine reuptake* can cause mydriasis (pupil dilation), sweating, tachycardia, early hypertension, myoclonus, and hyperreflexia. Furthermore, cyclic antidepressants *block sodium channels*, which slow conduction velocity, prolong repolarization, and depress myocardial contractility, potentially leading to heart blocks, bradycardia, and widening of the QRS complex. Finally, *potassium channel blockade* can result in QT interval prolongation and, in rare cases, Torsade de pointes [19].

3.2.2 Clinical features

Cyclic antidepressant toxicity symptoms can range from moderate antimuscarinic effects to severe cardiac toxicity, and they usually manifest within 2 hours of administration. The symptoms include excessive reflexes (hyperreflexia), muscular jerks (myoclonus), ataxia, slurred speech, lethargy, disorientation, and a fast heartbeat (sinus tachycardia). Symptoms of severe poisoning often appear 6 hours after intake and include ventricular tachycardia, low blood pressure, respiratory depression, unconsciousness, delays in cardiac conduction, and convulsions [20, 21].

ECG changes in cyclic antidepressant poisoning [22]:

- Sinus tachycardia.

- Right axis deviation of the terminal 40 milliseconds with positive terminal R wave in lead aVR and a negative S wave in lead I

- QRS prolongation (if the QRS complex is longer than 100 ms, the risk of seizures rises).

- QT and PR prolongation

- Brugada pattern is seen 10–15% (**Figure 2**)

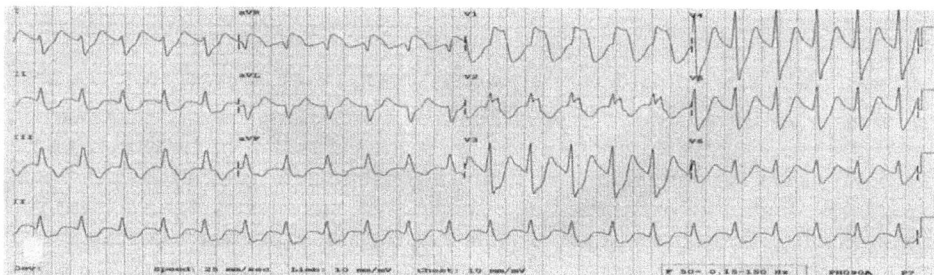

Figure 2
ECG changes in TCA toxicity [22].

3.2.3 Treatment

Treatment for cyclic antidepressant toxicity begins with supportive care, which includes securing the airway and administering intravenous fluids if the patient is hypotensive. Gastrointestinal decontamination with activated charcoal should be done within an hour of ingestion. If hypotension does not improve with IV fluids, vasopressors should be added. If the patient shows signs of cardiac conduction issues, ventricular arrhythmias, or persistent hypotension despite fluids, blood alkalinization with sodium bicarbonate should be started to maintain a blood pH of 7.50–7.55. For seizures, benzodiazepines are the first-line treatment; if seizures are resistant, phenobarbital (10–15 mg/kg) can be used. Certain medications are contraindicated in cyclic antidepressant toxicity, including Class I antiarrhythmics (such as lidocaine, phenytoin, and flecainide), Class III antiarrhythmics (such as amiodarone and sotalol), beta-blockers, calcium channel blockers, physostigmine, and flumazenil [23, 24].

3.3 Salicylate (aspirin) poisoning

Aspirin is a commonly used over-the-counter medication, frequently prescribed as an analgesic and antiplatelet agent for cardiovascular and cerebrovascular diseases. Due to its widespread availability and use, both accidental and intentional overdoses are common [25].

3.3.1 Mechanism of action

Aspirin works by inhibiting cyclooxygenase, which decreases the production of prostaglandins, prostacyclin, and thromboxane. This leads to platelet dysfunction and damage to the gastric mucosa. Aspirin also triggers the medulla's chemoreceptor trigger zone, which results in nausea and vomiting. Additionally, it triggers the medulla's respiratory center, resulting in respiratory alkalosis and hyperventilation. Moreover, aspirin causes metabolic acidosis by inhibiting the Krebs cycle and uncoupling oxidative phosphorylation [26].

3.3.2 Clinical features

Salicylate toxicity is divided into *acute* and *chronic* toxicities:

3.3.3 Acute toxicity

Acute toxicity presents with gastrointestinal, central nervous system (CNS), and metabolic symptoms. In the early stages, patients often experience gastric irritation, nausea, and vomiting, which are more common in acute poisoning cases. As salicylate levels in the CNS rise, symptoms such as tinnitus (ringing in the ears), reduced hearing, dizziness, and rapid breathing (hyperventilation) may occur. If the poisoning progresses, CNS effects can worsen, leading to agitation, hallucinations, delirium, seizures, and drowsiness. The metabolic effects of salicylate toxicity include uncoupling oxidative phosphorylation, which results in an elevated body temperature (a sign of severe toxicity) and a large anion gap metabolic acidosis. Severe cases can lead to renal failure, acute lung injury, and platelet dysfunction.

3.3.4 Chronic toxicity

Chronic salicylate toxicity, on the other hand, develops over a longer period, typically when a person unintentionally ingests more of the drug than their body can eliminate. This form of poisoning is more common in older individuals. The symptoms initially resemble those of acute toxicity, but they develop more slowly and are less severe. In elderly patients, chronic poisoning can easily be mistaken for conditions like sepsis, ketoacidosis, delirium, dementia, congestive heart failure, or respiratory failure. Delays in diagnosing chronic toxicity can lead to increased morbidity and mortality.

3.3.5 Treatment

Initial management of salicylate toxicity focuses on stabilizing airway, breathing, and circulation. Intubation should generally be avoided, as it can worsen the toxicity, but if it is required, the patient should receive adequate minute ventilation. If the patient is volume-depleted or experiencing acidosis, intravenous fluids should be administered. For early ingestions, gastrointestinal decontamination with activated charcoal may be helpful. Whole bowel irrigation (WBI) is recommended in cases of large or sustained ingestions, or when the medication is in sustained-release or enteric-coated form. Severe salicylate toxicity can be treated by alkalinizing the serum with sodium bicarbonate, aiming for a serum pH of around 7.5. In some cases, hemodialysis may be necessary, especially if there is clinical deterioration, severe acid–base imbalance, altered mental status, acute lung injury, failure of alkalinization methods, or renal failure [27–29].

3.4 Opioids poisoning

Opioid abuse has become a major medical and social issue globally. Over the past decade, there has been a significant rise in the number of opioid overdoses and related deaths. Opioids are a group of substances derived from opium, known for their pain-relieving and sedative properties. Opium itself is extracted from the poppy plant [30].

3.4.1 Mechanism of action

Opioids work by acting on three primary receptors in the body: μ (mu), κ (kappa), and δ (delta). When opioids bind to these receptors, they cause several effects, including pinpoint pupils (miosis), slowed breathing (respiratory depression), suppression of coughing, feelings of euphoria, and reduced movement in the digestive system (decreased GI motility).

3.4.2 Clinical features

The classic signs of opioid intoxication include a depressed mental state, slow breathing (low respiratory rate), and pinpoint (constricted) pupils. Other symptoms can include reduced bowel sounds, low blood pressure when standing (orthostatic hypotension), urinary retention, and localized skin reactions like hives (urticaria). In some cases, the pupils may appear normal, which can occur with toxins like meperidine, diphenoxylate, or propoxyphene, or when opioids are taken alongside other substances like sympathomimetics or anticholinergics (**Table 2**) [31, 32].

3.4.3 Treatment

The first crucial steps in treating opioid overdose are securing the airway and ensuring proper oxygenation and ventilation, typically using a bag-valve mask. It is important to check the patient's blood glucose levels as well. Then, administer naloxone at a dose of 0.4 mg IV. For non-opioid-dependent patients with mild respiratory depression, this dose is usually sufficient. However, for opioid-dependent individuals with minimal respiratory depression, administer a smaller dose of naloxone, such as 0.1 mg IV, as higher doses could trigger withdrawal symptoms. If the patient is experiencing apnea, near-apnea, or cyanosis, give naloxone 2 mg IV regardless of their drug use history, and repeat the dose every 3 minutes if necessary [31–33].

3.5 Sympathomimetic (cocaine) poisoning

Cocaine is made from the leaves of the coca plant and is one of the most potent sympathomimetics. It was initially employed in medicine in 1884 as a local anesthetic for eye-related procedures. In the United States, using cocaine is one of the most common causes of acute drug-related ED visits.

Opioids agent	Specific clinical feature
Dextromethorphan	Serotonin toxicity; at high doses
Loperamide	QRS and QT prolongation; Wide-complex tachycardia
Meperidine	Seizure, normal pupils size Serotonin syndrome (in combination with other agents)
Methadone	Long acting. QT prolongation, Torsade de Pointes
Oxycodone	QT interval prolongation
Tramadol	Seizure
Heroin	Acute lung injury

Table 2
Opioids with specific clinical features [31, 32].

3.5.1 Mechanism of action

Cocaine causes vasoconstriction in the cardiovascular system by stimulating alpha and adrenergic receptors by raising norepinephrine levels. It also prevents neuronal serotonin reuptake, which results in euphoria. Cocaine prolongs the QRS interval by blocking the sodium (Na+) channel [34, 35].

3.5.2 Clinical features

Cocaine poisoning can have vasoconstrictive and sympathomimetic effects on a number of systems, including the heart and central nervous system etc.).

- *Cardiovascu*lar: High blood pressure and dysrhythmias, such as tachycardia, sinus tachycardia, SVT, and AF, are common in individuals with cocaine poisoning. Moreover, QT interval prolongation and a rightward shift of the terminal part of the QRS complex are examples of ECG abnormalities. Patients may have myocarditis, cardiomyopathy, aortic and coronary artery dissection, and acute coronary syndromes (cocaine-associated acute coronary syndrome).

- CNS: A range of central nervous system symptoms, such as agitation, seizures, and coma, are seen in patients with cocaine poisoning.

- Pulmonary: Patients who use crack cocaine are more likely to get asthma, barotrauma, pneumonitis, and pulmonary hemorrhage.

- Gastrointestinal: Cocaine raises the risk of bleeding and ulcer perforation and can result in intestinal ischemia, ischemic colitis, and bowel necrosis.

- Renal: Rhabdomyolysis can result from cocaine poisoning, which can cause abrupt renal failure [36–38].

3.5.3 Treatment

The first stages of therapy include securing the airway and ensuring proper breathing. Benzodiazepines are used to sedate CNS symptoms (such as agitation or seizures). Rapid cooling is necessary for a patient suffering from hyperthermia. Phentolamine or a sodium nitroprusside infusion can be used to treat severe hypertension that is not responding to sedation (avoid B-ac blockers). Acute coronary syndrome caused by cocaine poisoning is treated with nitroglycerin and aspirin, and calcium channel blockers may also be used. Serum alkalinization by sodium bicarbonate is used to treat wide-complex tachycardia with cocaine toxicity; ensure that the serum pH does not rise over 7.55. When a patient has significant cocaine toxicity and resistant wide-complex tachycardia or cardiovascular instability, an intravenous lipid emulsion may be utilized [38].

- *Body packing*: swallowing smuggling packages or narcotic containers.

- Body stuffing: ingesting less medication out to fear of being arrested

3.6 Digitalis glycoside toxicity

Cardiac glycosides have been used for heart failure treatment for centuries, with their presence in plants such as foxglove, lily of the valley, and oleander. Digoxin is still a commonly used digitalis derivative for the treatment of congestive heart failure and atrial fibrillation [38].

3.6.1 Mechanism of action

During cardiac repolarization, digoxin inhibits Na+/K + -ATPase, which raises intracellular sodium and lowers intracellular potassium. This leads to an increase in intracellular calcium concentration, producing a positive inotropic effect. Additionally, digoxin enhances automaticity and shortens repolarization intervals in the atria and ventricles [39].

3.6.2 Clinical features

Toxicity from digoxin can be classified as acute or chronic:

- *Acute toxicity*: It typically results from accidental or intentional overdose and presents with nausea, vomiting, nonspecific abdominal pain, headache, and dizziness. Severe cases can progress to confusion, coma, bradyarrhythmias, atrioventricular (AV) block, supraventricular tachyarrhythmias, and hyperkalemia. A hallmark feature is xanthopsia, where patients perceive yellow-green halos around objects, though the most common visual disturbance is nonspecific color perception changes. Serum digoxin levels are significantly elevated [40, 41].

- Chronic toxicity: It is more common in elderly patients and often results from drug interactions (e.g., with calcium channel blockers, amiodarone, betablockers, or diuretics) or impaired renal clearance. Unlike acute toxicity, chronic digoxin toxicity prominently features CNS symptoms such as weakness, fatigue, confusion, or delirium. Ventricular arrhythmias are frequently observed. Serum potassium levels can be normal or decreased, with only slight elevations in serum digoxin levels [40–43].

3.6.3 Treatment

Supportive care is the cornerstone of management, including airway stabilization, ventilation support, and IV fluid resuscitation for hypotension. Activated charcoal is beneficial for early acute ingestion. Atropine is administered for symptomatic bradycardia. Digoxin-specific antibody fragments (digoxin-Fab) serve as an antidote in cases of life-threatening arrhythmias unresponsive to standard treatment or hyperkalemia exceeding 6 mEq/L. Digoxin-Fab dosage requirements are determined by total-body digoxin burden, which may be calculated from blood levels or the amount consumed [44]. Every digoxin-Fab vial neutralizes around 0.5 milligrams of digoxin. An empirical dosage of ten vials may be given if the amount consumed is unclear. Hyperkalemia is managed with insulin, dextrose, and sodium bicarbonate. The use of calcium salts remains controversial due to historical reports of increased ventricular arrhythmias and mortality [40, 41].

3.7 Beta-blocker toxicity

Beta-adrenergic antagonists, commonly known as beta-blockers, have been widely used for over three decades in the management of cardiovascular, neurological, and ophthalmologic conditions. However, beta-blocker overdose is associated with significant morbidity and mortality [17].

3.7.1 Mechanism of action

Beta receptors are categorized into three types based on their location and function: (see **Table 3**).

- *Beta-1 (B1)*: Found in the myocardium, kidneys, and eyes, these receptors enhance inotropy, chronotropy, and renin release. Beta-1 blockade results in reduced myocardial contractility, heart rate, and renin secretion.

- Beta-2 (B2): Located in bronchial smooth muscle, skeletal muscle, the liver, and vasculature, these receptors promote bronchodilation, uterine relaxation, increased contraction force, and vasodilation. Beta-2 antagonism leads to bronchospasm, inhibition of glycogenolysis and gluconeogenesis, and minimal vasoconstriction.

- Beta-3 (B3): Present in adipose tissue and skeletal muscle, these receptors stimulate lipolysis and thermogenesis. Beta-3 blockade results in the inhibition of these processes.

Beta-blockers are classified as either selective (targeting beta-1 receptors) or nonselective (affecting both beta-1 and beta-2 receptors). These drugs work by competitively inhibiting beta receptors, reducing intracellular cyclic adenosine monophosphate (cAMP) levels. Selective beta-1 blockade primarily impacts myocardial contractility, pacemaker automaticity, and AV node conduction, whereas nonselective beta-blockers have systemic effects, including bronchoconstriction and impaired gluconeogenesis. Lipophilic beta-blockers, such as propranolol, cross the blood–brain barrier rapidly, leading to neurological symptoms like seizures and delirium [45, 46].

	Location	Action	Antagonism
B1	Myocardium Kidney Eye	Increases inotropy Increases chronotropy Stimulates renin release	Decreases inotropy Decreases chronotropy Inhibits renin release
B2	Bronchial smooth muscle Skeletal muscle Liver Vascular	Bronchodilation Relaxes uterus Increases force of contraction Stimulates glycogenolysis & gluconeogenesis Vasodilation	Causes bronchospasm Inhibits glycogenolysis and gluconeogenesis Minimal vasoconstriction
B3	Adipose tissue Skeletal muscle	Stimulates lipolysis Stimulates thermogenesis	Inhibits lipolysis Inhibits thermogenesis

Table 3
Beta receptor: Locations and actions.

3.7.2 Clinical manifestations

Beta-blocker toxicity primarily affects the cardiovascular system, resulting in bradycardia and hypotension. Bradycardia arises from sinus node suppression or conduction abnormalities. However, beta-blockers with partial agonist activity may initially present with hypertension and tachycardia. Some beta-blockers, such as sotalol, also block potassium channels, leading to QT interval prolongation and potential arrhythmias.

CNS and pulmonary involvement may include delirium, coma, seizures (more common with lipophilic beta-blockers like propranolol), bronchospasm, and hypoglycemia [46, 47].

3.7.3 Treatment

Management includes early GI decontamination with activated charcoal if the patient presents within 1 hour of ingestion. The primary focus of treatment is restoring perfusion to critical organs by increasing cardiac output. This can be achieved through:

1. Fluid resuscitation

2. Glucagon administration (3–10 mg IV) to enhance myocardial contractility

3. Vasopressors (e.g., epinephrine) for refractory hypotension

4. High-dose insulin-glucose therapy (1 unit/kg IV bolus of insulin)

5. Intravenous lipid emulsion therapy is considered in severe toxicity cases unresponsive to standard treatments. In cases refractory to pharmacological therapy, advanced interventions such as hemodialysis, hemoperfusion, cardiac pacing, or intra-aortic balloon pump placement may be required. Wide QRS-interval arrhythmias caused by sodium channel inhibition caused by beta-blockers are treated with sodium bicarbonate (2–3 mEq/kg IV over 1–2 minutes) [48, 49].

3.8 Calcium channel blocker toxicity

Many cardiovascular diseases, including hypertension, coronary artery disease, and arrhythmias, are treated with calcium channel blockers (CCBs). Due to their widespread prescription, toxicity from these drugs is common. CCBs are available in immediate-release and extended-release formulations [17].

3.8.1 Mechanism of action

CCBs are classified into two primary categories based on their predominant physiological effects:

- *Dihydropyridines (e.g., amlodipi*ne, nifedipine): Primarily act on L-type calcium channels in vascular smooth muscle, leading to vasodilation and reflex tachycardia.

- Non-dihydropyridines (e.g., verapamil, diltiazem): Preferentially block L-type calcium channels in the myocardium, reducing cardiac contractility and causing bradycardia.

In overdose, dihydropyridines primarily result in vasodilatory shock, whereas non-dihydropyridines can lead to significant myocardial depression and conduction abnormalities [50].

3.8.2 Clinical manifestations

The cardiovascular system is the primary target of CCB toxicity. Patients often present with hypotension, bradycardia, and, in the case of dihydropyridine toxicity, reflex tachycardia. Verapamil and diltiazem overdoses typically result in sinus brady-cardia. Unlike beta-blockers, CCBs generally do not have a primary effect on the CNS or pulmonary system. CNS manifestations such as seizures, delirium, and coma are secondary to poor organ perfusion. Severe cases may develop cardiogenic pulmonary edema and acute lung injury [47].

3.8.3 Treatment

1. Initial management includes securing the airway and stabilizing ventilation and circulation. Decontamination with activated charcoal is effective if administered within 1 hour of ingestion, while whole-bowel irrigation is recommended for extended-release CCB ingestions.

2. IV fluid resuscitation for hypotension

3. Calcium chloride or calcium gluconate to counteract myocardial depression

4. Glucagon (3–10 mg IV) if initial measures fail

5. Vasopressors (e.g., norepinephrine) if unresponsive to fluids and calcium

For refractory cases, high-dose insulin-glucose therapy can improve cardiac contractility. If hypotension persists despite maximal medical therapy, lipid emulsion therapy may be considered. Circulatory support measures such as intra-aortic balloon pump placement may be used in severe cases [48, 49, 51].

3.9 Carbon monoxide poisoning

Carbon monoxide (CO) is a colorless, odorless, tasteless, and nonirritating gas. Common sources of exposure include automotive exhaust, fuel-powered heaters, wood or coal-burning stoves, structure fires, and gasoline-powered generators. The increasing use of wood stoves, space heaters, and charcoal indoors during the winter increases the risk of CO poisoning.

3.9.1 Mechanism of action

CO has a 200-fold higher affinity for hemoglobin than oxygen and diffuses quickly across the pulmonary capillary membrane. This binding forms carboxyhemoglobin, which impairs oxygen delivery to tissues and shifts the oxyhemoglobin dissociation curve to the left, reducing oxygen release at the tissue level [51].

3.9.2 Clinical features

Symptoms of CO poisoning vary based on exposure severity:

- *Mild to* moderate: Headache, nausea, and dizziness

- Severe: Confusion, seizures, and coma

- Cardiovascular complications: Myocardial injury, life-threatening arrhythmias

- Neurological sequelae: Delayed neuropsychiatric syndrome (DNS), which presents with cognitive impairments, movement disorders, and focal neurologic deficits

Standard pulse oximetry cannot distinguish carboxyhemoglobin from oxyhemoglobin, making it unreliable for diagnosis. Carboxyhemoglobin levels must be measured *via* arterial blood gas analysis [52–55].

3.9.3 Treatment

After airway stabilization, the primary treatment is 100% oxygen *via* a non-rebreather mask or mechanical ventilation if necessary. Oxygen therapy reduces the half-life of carboxyhemoglobin from approximately 250–320 minutes in room air to 90 minutes with 100% oxygen.
Hyperbaric oxygen (HBO) therapy is recommended in specific cases, including:

1. Pregnant patients with carboxyhemoglobin levels >15%

2. Nonpregnant patients with carboxyhemoglobin levels >25%

3. Evidence of acute myocardial ischemia

4. Severe metabolic acidosis [56].

3.10 Iron toxicity

Iron tablets are commonly found in households, particularly those with children and pregnant women. Their candy-like appearance, bright color, and sugar coating make them attractive to children, raising the risk of accidental ingestion [57].

3.10.1 Mechanism of action

Excessive iron exerts corrosive effects on the gastrointestinal tract and has cytotoxic actions, particularly in the liver, leading to hepatocellular necrosis. Additionally, iron has cardiotoxic effects, acting as a negative inotrope and inhibiting thrombin activity, resulting in coagulopathy. These effects contribute to metabolic acidosis [58].

3.10.2 Clinical features

Iron poisoning occurs in five stages:

1. Within 6 hours: Vomiting, hematemesis, diarrhea, abdominal pain, drowsiness, and irritability. Severe poisoning may cause coma, seizures, rapid breathing, and hypotension.

2. 6–48 hours: Symptoms may improve during a latent phase, leading to misinterpretation as recovery.

3. 12–48 hours: Shock, fever, bleeding, jaundice, liver failure, metabolic acidosis, and seizures can occur.

4. 2–5 days: Liver failure, coagulopathy, hypoglycemia, and coma.

5. 2–5 weeks: Gastrointestinal scarring may cause bowel obstruction [59, 60].

3.10.3 Treatment

- Initial management includes stabilizing the airway, breathing, and circulation.

- An abdominal X-ray may confirm the presence of iron tablets.

- Whole bowel irrigation is recommended for patients with large ingestions, especially of sustained-release formulations.

- Activated charcoal is ineffective in binding iron.

- Asymptomatic patients require observation for 6 hours.

- Serum iron levels <300–350 mcg/dL allow for safe discharge.

- Chelation therapy with deferoxamine is indicated for:

- Serum iron >350 mcg/dL with symptoms

- Serum iron >500 mcg/dL regardless of symptoms

- In severe cases with persistent metabolic acidosis or hemodynamic instability, deferoxamine therapy should not be delayed. Hemodialysis is ineffective in removing iron but may be considered in cases of acute renal failure to facilitate removal of the iron-deferoxamine complex [61, 62].

3.11 Toxic alcohol poisoning

Toxic alcohols, including methanol, ethylene glycol (EG), and isopropanol, are fewer common causes of poisoning but can result in severe morbidity and mortality if not promptly diagnosed and managed [63, 64].

3.11.1 Mechanism of action and clinical features

- *Meth*anol: It is found in windshield wiper fluid, paint removers, and deicing solutions. In the liver, methanol metabolized to formaldehyde and subsequently to formic acid, which inhibits mitochondrial cytochrome c, leading to lactic acidosis and optic nerve toxicity. Classic signs include severe anion gap metabolic acidosis, visual disturbances, and altered mental status. Pancreatitis may also occur.

- Ethylene glycol: It is present in radiator antifreeze and metal cleaners. It is metabolized to glycolic and oxalic acid, leading to metabolic acidosis, hypocalcemia, and calcium oxalate crystal deposition in the kidneys, resulting in renal failure. Neurological symptoms include coma, seizures, and muscle spasms.

- Isopropanol: It is found in solvents, disinfectants, and hand sanitizers. It is metabolized to acetone and typically does not cause metabolic acidosis. Clinical features include inebriation, cerebellar signs, and hemorrhagic gastritis [64–70].

3.11.2 Investigations

1. Osmolar gap >10 mOsm/kg suggests toxicity from ethylene glycol, methanol, or isopropanol.

2. High anion gap metabolic acidosis is seen in methanol and ethylene glycol poisoning.

3. Hypoglycemia may occur with isopropanol, whereas hyperglycemia and hypocalcemia can occur in methanol and ethylene glycol poisonings, respectively.

4. Urinary calcium oxalate crystals are indicative of ethylene glycol intoxication [71, 72].

3.11.3 Treatment

- Early stabilization includes airway management, respiratory support, and correction of metabolic derangements.

- Fomepizole: Inhibits alcohol dehydrogenase, preventing the formation of toxic metabolites from methanol and ethylene glycol.

- Hemodialysis: Indicated in cases of severe metabolic acidosis, refractory hypotension, or end-organ damage.

- Vitamin therapy: Folic or folinic acid for methanol poisoning to facilitate detoxification of formic acid. Pyridoxine and thiamine for ethylene glycol toxicity to promote metabolism to nontoxic metabolites [73–76].

3.12 Organophosphate poisoning

Organophosphates (OPs) are widely used in insecticides for agricultural and domestic purposes and serve as the primary toxic agents in nerve gases like sarin. OP pesticide self-poisoning is a significant public health issue, particularly in rural regions of Asia [77].

3.12.1 Mechanism of action

The most severe cases of OP poisoning occur *via* ingestion, while dermal absorption and inhalation of sprays are less likely to result in critical toxicity. OPs exert their toxic effects by inhibiting acetylcholinesterase, leading to an excessive accumulation of acetylcholine at muscarinic, nicotinic, and central nervous system (CNS) receptors.

3.12.2 Clinical features

Patients present with a cholinergic crisis within 4 hours of exposure, which may include:

- *Muscarinic effects*: Bronchospasm, pinpoint pupils, bradycardia, hypotension, excessive salivation, lacrimation, urination, diarrhea, vomiting, and profuse sweating.

- *Nicotinic effects*: Muscle fasciculations, cramps, weakness, tachycardia, and hypertension.

- *CNS effects*: Delirium, seizures, and coma.

- *Respiratory failure*: The primary cause of mortality in severe OP poisoning due to bronchorrhea and respiratory muscle paralysis.

Toxicity may persist due to irreversible binding of OPs to cholinesterase enzymes, known as "aging." This process stabilizes the enzyme-inhibitor complex, leading to prolonged symptoms. The "intermediate syndrome" occurs 24–96 hours post-exposure, characterized by cranial nerve involvement, proximal muscle weakness, and variable recovery over days to weeks [78].

3.12.3 Treatment

- Medical management requires immediate decontamination, administration of antidotes, and supportive care. Healthcare providers must wear protective clothing to prevent secondary contamination.

- Decontamination: Remove contaminated clothing and perform a thorough wash in a designated decontamination area.

- Atropine: Acts as a muscarinic antagonist to counteract cholinergic effects. Doses are titrated to the resolution of bronchorrhea.

- Oximes (Pralidoxime): Reactivates acetylcholinesterase by cleaving the phosphate bond if administered early, preventing aging of the enzyme.

- Respiratory Support: Mechanical ventilation may be required in cases of respiratory failure.

- Observation: Patients must be monitored for recurrent toxicity due to lipophilic OP redistribution [79, 80].

4. Conclusion

Managing poisoned patients in the emergency department poses unique challenges due to difficulties in obtaining an accurate history and identifying the specific toxic agent. A structured approach begins with resuscitation, stabilization of the airway, breathing, and circulation, and early decontamination when appropriate.

A thorough physical examination and recognition of toxidromes can aid in diagnosis. Most cases require laboratory tests, including complete blood count, electrolyte panels, kidney function assessments, and specific drug levels. Paracetamol levels should be obtained in all suspected overdose cases.

Symptomatic treatment remains the foundation of toxicology management, supplemented by antidotes in specific poisonings. Coordination with local poison control centers is crucial for up-to-date guidance and advanced interventions.

Author details

Ehab Aki*, Mohammed Abdurabu and Mohamed Elgassim
Hamad Medical Corporation, Doha, Qatar

*Address all correspondence to: akiehab2004@gmail.com

IntechOpen

References

[1] Warner M, Chen LH, Makuc DM, et al. Drug Poisoning Deaths in the United States, 1980-2008. NCHS Data Brief, no. 81. Hyattsville, MD: National Center for Health Statistics; 2011

[2] Liu Q, Zhou L, Zheng N, et al. Poisoning deaths in China: Type and prevalence detected at the Tongji forensic medical Center in Hubei. Forensic Science International. 2009;**193**:88

[3] Erickson TB, Thompson TM, Lu JJ. The approach to the patient with an unknown overdose. Emergency Medicine Clinics of North America. 2007;**25**:249

[4] Greene S et al. . In: Tintinalli JE et al., editors. General Management of Poisoned Patients. Tintinalli's Emergency Medicine: A Comprehensive Study Guide. 8e ed. New York, NY: McGraw-Hill; 2016

[5] Mofenson HC, Greensher J. The nontoxic ingestion. Paediatric Clinics of North America. 1970;**17**(3):583-590

[6] Manoguerra AS, Cobaugh DJ. Guidelines for the Management of Poisoning Consensus Panel: Guideline on the use of ipecac syrup in the out-of-hospital management of ingested poisons. Clinical Toxicology (Philadelphia, Pa.). 2005;**43**:1

[7] Adams BK, Mann MD, Aboo A, et al. Prolonged gastric emptying half-time and gastric hypomotility after drug overdose. The American Journal of Emergency Medicine. 2004;**22**:548

[8] Position paper: Whole bowel irrigation. Journal of Toxicology. Clinical Toxicology. 2004;**42**:843

[9] Bunchorntavakul C, Reddy KR. Acetaminophen-related hepatotoxicity. Clinics in Liver Disease. 2013;**17**:587

[10] Watson WA, Litovitz TL, Klein-Schwartz W, et al. 2003 annual report of the American Association of Poison Control Centers Toxic Exposure Surveillance System. The American Journal of Emergency Medicine. 2004;**22**:335

[11] Manyike PT, Kharasch ED, Kalhorn TF, Slattery JT. Contribution of CYP2E1 and CYP3A to acetaminophen reactive metabolite formation. Clinical Pharmacology and Therapeutics. 2000;**67**:275

[12] Fontana RJ. Acute liver failure including acetaminophen overdose. The Medical Clinics of North America. 2008;**92**:761

[13] Waring WS, Stephen AF, Malkowska AM, Robinson OD. Acute acetaminophen overdose is associated with dose-dependent hypokalaemia: A prospective study of 331 patients. Basic & Clinical Pharmacology & Toxicology. 2008;**102**:325

[14] Bernal W et al. Blood lactate as an early predictor outcome in paracetamol-induced acute liver failure: A cohort study. Lancet. 2002;**359**:558-563

[15] Harrison PM, Wendon JA, Gimson AES, et al. Improvement by acetylcysteine of hemodynamic and oxygen transfort in fulminant hepatic failure. The New England Journal of Medicine. 1991;**324**:1852-1857

[16] Rumack-Matthew H. Acetaminophen poisoning and toxicity. Pediatrics. 1975;**55**:871

[17] Mowry JB, Spyker DA, Cantilena LR, McMillan H, Ford M. Annual report of the American Association of Poison Control Centers' National Poison Data System (NPDS): 31th annual report. Clinical Toxicology (Philadelphia, Pa.). 2013;**52**(1032):2014

[18] Furukawa TA, McGuire H, Barbui C. Meta-analysis of effects and side effects of low dosage tricyclic antidepressants in depression: Systematic review. BMJ. 2002;**325**:991

[19] Fanoe S, Kristensen D, Fink-Jensena, et al. Risk of arrhythmia induced by psychotropic medications: A proposal for clinical management. European Heart Journal. 2014;**35**:1306

[20] White N, Litovitz T, Clancy C. Suicidal antidepressant overdoses: A comparative analysis by antidepressant type. Journal of Medical Toxicology. 2008;**4**:238

[21] Bateman DN. Tricyclic antidepressant poisoning, central nervous system effects and management. Toxicological Reviews. 2005;**24**:181

[22] ECG Changes in TCA Toxicity; 2024. Available from: https://litfl.com/tricyclic-overdose-sodium-channel-blocker-toxicity/

[23] Teece S, Hogg L. Towards evidence based emergency medicine: Best BETs from the Manchester Royal Infirmary. Glucagon in tricyclic overdose. Emergency Medicine Journal. 2003;**20**:264

[24] Lo Vecchio F. Cyclic Antidepressants. In: Tintinalli's Emergency Medicine: A Comprehensive Study Guide. 8e ed. New York, NY: McGraw-Hill; 2016

[25] Herres J, Ryan D, Salzman M. Delayed salicylate toxicity with

undetectable initial levels after large-dose aspirin ingestion. The American Journal of Emergency Medicine. 2009;**27**:1173.e1

[26] O'Malley GF. Emergency department management of the salicylate-poisoned patient. Emergency Medicine Clinics of North America. 2007;**25**:333

[27] Greenberg MI, Hendrickson RG, Hofman M. Deleterious effects of endotracheal intubation in salicylate poisoning. Annals of Emergency Medicine. 2003;**41**:583

[28] Thanacoody R, Caravati EM, Troutman B, et al. Position paper update: Whole bowel irrigation for gastrointestinal decontamination of overdose patients. Clinical Toxicology (Philadelphia, Pa.). 2015;**53**:5

[29] Juurlink DN, Gosselin S, Kielstein JT, et al. Extracorporeal treatment for salicylate poisoning: Systematic review and recommendations from the EXTRIP workgroup. Annals of Emergency Medicine. 2015;**66**:165

[30] Watson WA, Litovitz TL, Rodgers GC Jr, et al. 2004 annual report of the American Association of Poison Control Centers Toxic Exposure Surveillance System. The American Journal of Emergency Medicine. 2005;**23**:589

[31] Sporer KA. Acute heroin overdose. Annals of Internal Medicine. 1999;**130**:584

[32] Burillo-Putze G, Miro O. Opioids. In: Tintinalli's Emergency Medicine: A Comprehensive Study Guide. 8e ed. New York, NY: McGraw-Hill; 2016

[33] Dowling J, Isbister GK, Kirkpatrick CM, Naidoo D, Graudins A. Population pharmacokinetics of intravenous, intramuscular, and

intranasal naloxone in human volunteers. Therapeutic Drug Monitoring. 2008;**30**:490

[34] Hoffman RS, Kaplan JL, Hung OL, Goldfrank LR. Ecgonine methyl ester protects against cocaine lethality in mice. Journal of Toxicology. Clinical Toxicology. 2004;**42**:349

[35] Ritz MC, Lamb RJ, Goldberg SR, Kuhar MJ. Cocaine receptors on dopamine transporters are related to self-administration of cocaine. Science. 1987;**237**:1219

[36] Lange RA, Cigarroa RG, Flores ED, et al. Potentiation of cocaine-induced coronary vasoconstriction by beta-adrenergic blockade. Annals of Internal Medicine. 1990;**112**:897

[37] Osborn HH, Tang M, Bradley K, et al. New onset bronchospasm or recrudescence of asthma associated with cocaine abuse. Academic Emergency Medicine. 1997;**4**:689

[38] Prosser JM, Perrone J. Cocaine and amphetamines. In: Tintinalli's Emergency Medicine: A Comprehensive Study Guide. 8e ed. New York, NY: McGraw-Hill; 2016

[39] Eichhorn EJ, Gheorghiade M. Digoxin. Progress in Cardiovascular Diseases. 2002;**44**:251-266

[40] Smith TW, Digitalis. Mechanisms of action and clinical use. The New England Journal of Medicine. 1988;**318**:358

[41] Kanji S, MacLean RD. Cardiac glycoside toxicity: More than 200 years and counting. Critical Care Clinics. 2012;**28**:527

[42] Bhatia SJ. Digitalis toxicity—Turning over a new leaf? The Western Journal of Medicine. 1986;**145**:74

[43] Roberts DM, Buckley NA. Antidotes for acute cardenolide (cardiac glycoside) poisoning. Cochrane Database of Systematic Reviews. 2006;**4**:CD005490

[44] Antman EM, Wenger TL, Butler VP Jr, Haber E, Smith TW. Treatment of 150 cases of life-threatening digitalis intoxication with digoxin-specific fab antibody fragments. Final report of a multicentre study. Circulation. 1990;**81**:1744

[45] Hack JB, Woody JH, Lewis DE, Brewer K, Meggs WJ. The effect of calcium chloride in treating hyperkalemia due to acute digoxin toxicity in a porcine model. Journal of Toxicology. Clinical Toxicology. 2004;**42**:337

[46] Samuels TL, Uncles DR, Willers JW, et al. Logging the potential for intravenous lipid emulsion in propranolol and other lipophilic drug overdoses. Anaesthesia. 2011;**66**:221

[47] DeWitt CR, Waksman JC. Pharmacology, pathophysiology, and management of calcium channel blocker and beta-blocker toxicity. Toxicological Reviews. 2004;**23**:223

[48] Kerns W. Management of beta-adrenergic blocker and calcium channel antagonist toxicity. Emergency Medicine Clinics of North America. 2007;**25**:309

[49] Wax PM, Erdman AR, Chyka PA, et al. Beta-blocker ingestion: An evidence-based consensus guideline for out-of-hospital management. Clinical Toxicology (Philadelphia, Pa.). 2005;**43**:131

[50] Vucinić S, Joksović D, Jovanović D, et al. Factors influencing the degree and outcome of acute beta-blockers poisoning. Vojnosanitetski Pregled. 2000;**57**:619

[51] Jang DH, Spyres MB, Fox L, Manini AF. Toxin-induced cardiovascular failure. Emergency Medicine Clinics of North America. 2014;**32**:79

[52] Hardy KR, Thom SR. Pathophysiology and treatment of carbon monoxide poisoning. Journal of Toxicology. Clinical Toxicology. 1994;**32**:613

[53] Kao LW, Nañagas KA. Carbon monoxide poisoning. Emergency Medicine Clinics of North America. 2004;**22**:985

[54] Thom SR, Taber RL, Mendiguren II, et al. Delayed neuropsychologic sequelae after carbon monoxide poisoning: Prevention by treatment with hyperbaric oxygen. Annals of Emergency Medicine. 1995;**25**:474

[55] Henry CR, Satran D, Lindgren B, et al. Myocardial injury and long-term mortality following moderate to severe carbon monoxide poisoning. JAMA. 2006;**295**:398

[56] Bozeman WP, Myers RA, Barish RA. Confirmation of the pulse oximetry gap in carbon monoxide poisoning. Annals of Emergency Medicine. 1997;**30**:608

[57] Ziser A, Shupak A, Halpern P, et al. Delayed hyperbaric oxygen treatment for acute carbon monoxide poisoning. British Medical Journal (Clinical Research Ed.). 1984;**289**:960

[58] Morris CC. Paediatrics iron poisonings in the United States. Southern Medical Journal. 2000;**93**:352

[59] Anderson GJ, Wang F. Essential but toxic: Controlling the flux of iron in the body. Clinical and Experimental Pharmacology & Physiology. 2012;**39**:719

[60] Singhi SC, Baranwal AK, Jayashree M. Acute iron poisoning: Clinical picture, intensive care needs and outcome. Indian Paediatric. 2003;**40**:1177

[61] Robertson A, Tenenbein M. Hepatotoxicity in acute iron poisoning. Human & Experimental Toxicology. 2005;**24**:559

[62] Manoguerra AS, Erdman AR, Booze LL, et al. Iron ingestion: An evidence-based consensus guideline for out-of-hospital management. Clinical Toxicology (Philadelphia, Pa.). 2005;**43**:553

[63] Baranwal AK, Singhi SC. Acute iron poisoning: management guidelines. Indian Podiatric. 2003;**40**:534

[64] Jammalamadaka D, Raissi S. Ethylene glycol, methanol and isopropyl alcohol intoxication. The American Journal of the Medical Sciences. 2010;**339**:276-281

[65] Burkhart KK, Kulig KW. The other alcohols—Methanol, ethylene glycol, and isopropanol. Emergency Medicine Clinics of North America. 1990;**8**:913-928

[66] Barceloux DG, Bond GR, Krenzelok EP, et al. American Academy of clinical toxicology practice guidelines on the treatment of methanol poisoning. Clinical Toxicology. 2002;**40**:415-446

[67] Onder F, Ilker S, Kansu T, et al. Acute blindness and putaminal necrosis in methanol intoxication. International Ophthalmology. 1999;**22**:81-84

[68] Hantson P, Mahieu P. Pancreatic injury following acute methanol poisoning. Clinical Toxicology. 2000;**38**:297-303

[69] Eder AF, McGrath CM, et al. Methylene glycol poisoning:

Toxicokinetic and analytical factors affecting laboratory diagnosis Shaw. Clinical Chemistry. 1998;**44**(1):168-177

[70] Wolfson AB et al. Ethylene glycol. In: Harwood-Nuss' Clinical Practice of Emergency Medicine. Philadelphia: Lippincott Williams and Wilkins Co.; 2005. pp. 1454-1458

[71] Jacobsen D, Bredesen JE, Eide I, et al. Anion and osmolal gaps in the diagnosis of methanol and ethylene glycol poisoning. Acta Medica Scandinavica. 1982;**22**:17-20

[72] Hassanian-Moghaddam H, Pajoumand A, Dadgar SM, Shadnia S. Prognostic factors In methanol poisoning. Human & Experimental Toxicology. 2007;**26**:583-586

[73] Wiener SW. Toxic alcohols. In: Nelson LS et al., editors. Goldfrank's Toxicologic Emergencies. 10th ed. McGrawHill; 2015. pp. 1346-1358

[74] Mégarbane B, Borron SW, Baud FJ. Intensive Care Medicine. 2005;**31**:189

[75] Lepik KJ et al. Adverse drug events associated with the antidotes for methanol and ethylene glycol poisoning: A comparison of ethanol and fomepizole. Annals of Emergency Medicine. 2009;**53**(4):439-450

[76] Kraut JA. Ira Kurtz toxic alcohol ingestions: Clinical features, diagnosis, and management. CJASN. 2008;**3**:208-225

[77] Emmett M, Palmer BF. Serum osmolal gap. In: Forman JP, editor. UpToDate. Waltham, MA; 2016

[78] Hulse EJ, Davies JOJ, Simpson AJ, et al. Respiratory complications of organophosphorus nerve agent and insecticide poisoning. American Journal of Respiratory and Critical Care Medicine. 2014;**190**(12):1342-1354

[79] Wayne R. Diagnosis and treatment of poisoning due to pesticides. In: Hayes' Handbook of Pesticide Toxicology. Third ed. 2010

[80] Eddleston M, Singh S, Buckley N. Organophosphorus poisoning (acute). Clinical Evidence. 2005;**13**:1744-1755

Chapter 3

Paracetamol (Acetaminophen) Poisoning

Mutwakil Elbidairi

Abstract

Acetaminophen (APAP) is a commonly used medication for its antipyretic and analgesic properties, yet it is the leading cause of acute liver failure in the United States. This chapter explores the widespread use of APAP, the mechanisms underlying its toxic effects, and the clinical management of overdose cases. It discusses the pathophysiology of APAP metabolism, where the production of the toxic metabolite N-acetyl-p-benzoquinone imine (NAPQI) leads to hepatotoxicity when consumed in excessive doses. The chapter also outlines the various presentations of APAP toxicity, from acute single-dose poisoning to repeated supratherapeutic ingestion, emphasizing the importance of early intervention. Clinical management strategies, including the use of N-acetylcysteine (NAC) as an antidote, are highlighted to prevent severe outcomes. The chapter concludes with an overview of monitoring protocols and prognostic indicators, providing a comprehensive understanding of APAP overdose and its treatment.

Keywords: acetaminophen overdose, APAP toxicity, acute liver failure, N-acetylcysteine, hepatotoxicity

1. Introduction

Since its first clinical use in 1950, acetaminophen (N-acetyl-p-aminophenol, APAP) has remained a widely used antipyretic and analgesic. However, it is the leading cause of acute liver failure in the United States [1, 2], with unintentional poisoning slightly surpassing intentional overdose cases. This often occurs because individuals may not be aware of the potential dangers of APAP, leading to unintentional overdose through the consumption of multiple nonprescription drugs containing APAP or the misuse of combination opioid/APAP analgesics. According to data from the Toxic Exposure Surveillance System, APAP ingestion ranks fourth among fatal ingestions [2]. Acetaminophen poisoning is one of the most frequent causes of medication-related poisoning and death, resulting from either acute or repeated supratherapeutic ingestion. Management of an acetaminophen-poisoned patient involves stabilization, decontamination, and the administration of acetylcysteine, a specific antidote. The decision to use acetylcysteine or perform gastrointestinal decontamination is based on the patient's symptoms, timing and duration of exposure, and serum acetaminophen and aminotransferase levels [3].

IntechOpen

The antipyretic and analgesic effects of APAP are thought to be mediated through central inhibition of the COX-2 enzyme involved in prostaglandin synthesis [4]. APAP is rapidly absorbed from the gastrointestinal tract, with peak serum concentrations observed between 30 minutes and 2 hours [5, 6].

Experts consider a potentially toxic ingestion of APAP to be greater than 150 mg/kg or 7.5 g within a 4-hour period. The FDA recommends a maximum daily dose of 4 grams [6, 7].

2. Pathophysiology of paracetamol overdose

The metabolism of acetaminophen (APAP) is well understood (see **Figure 1**). In the liver, APAP is primarily converted into non-toxic metabolites through glucuronidation (40–67%) and sulfation (20–46%) [5, 6]. A small portion is excreted unchanged by the kidneys. Both APAP-glucuronide and APAP-sulfate are eliminated via renal excretion. A minor fraction of APAP is metabolized by the cytochrome P450 system to produce N-acetyl-p-benzoquinone imine (NAPQI), a highly reactive compound that can oxidize and damage essential cellular proteins. Since NAPQI is predominantly formed in the liver, hepatotoxicity is a key feature of APAP poisoning [7, 8].

At therapeutic doses, the small amount of NAPQI produced is neutralized by conjugation with reduced glutathione (GSH), as shown in **Figure 1**, a crucial tripeptide that, in an NADPH-dependent reaction, helps detoxify oxidants like NAPQI. However, in cases of large APAP overdoses, the usual metabolic pathways become saturated, leading to the depletion of endogenous glutathione. Consequently, NAPQI remains unmetabolized, resulting in toxicity. This manifests microscopically as hepatic necrosis, especially near the terminal hepatic vein, where cytochrome P450 enzymes are concentrated. Individuals with upregulated CYP450 2E1, such as alcoholics, are particularly vulnerable to liver failure from APAP use [7, 8].

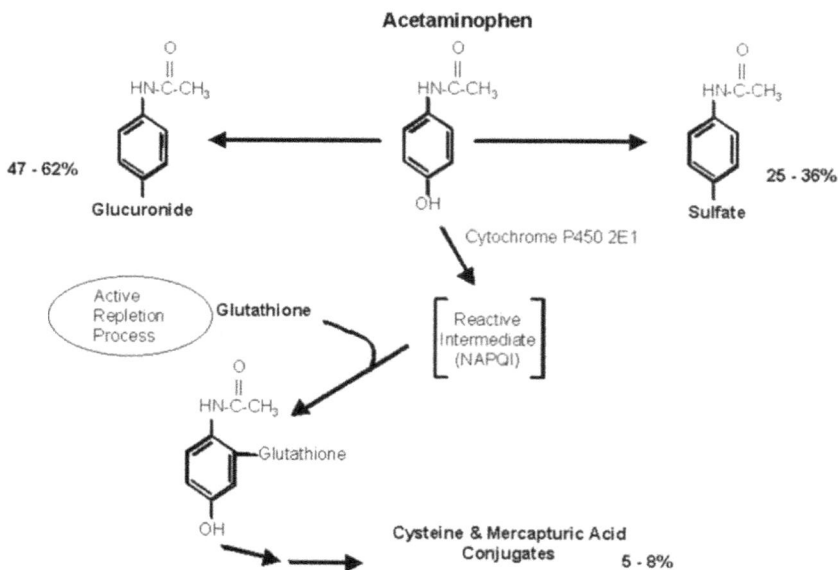

Figure 1.
Metabolism of APAP.

3. Toxic ingestion

3.1 Acute single-dose poisoning

Toxic dose: ≥150 mg/kg or ≥ 7.5 g in adults and adolescents.

3.2 Repeated supratherapeutic ingestion

- Children (<6 years):

  o ≥150 mg/kg/day for 2 days or longer.

  o ≥100 mg/kg/day for 3 days or longer.

- Adolescents and Adults (≥6 years):

  o ≥10 g/day or 200 mg/kg/day (whichever is less) over 24 hours.

  o ≥6 g/day or 150 mg/kg/day for 48 hours or more.

Risk factors: chronic alcohol use, fasting states, or concurrent use of CYP450-inducing drugs like isoniazid.

3.3 Sustained-release preparations

- Toxic dose: ≥150 mg/kg or ≥ 7.5 g.

- Recommendations: Measure serum paracetamol levels at 4 hours post-ingestion and repeat 4 hours later. Start N-acetylcysteine (NAC) if either value is above the nomogram line.

4. Clinical manifestations of APAP toxicity

Clinicians categorize acetaminophen (APAP) toxicity into four distinct stages, each with unique clinical presentations. *Stage I* (0–24 hours post-ingestion) often involves nonspecific symptoms or none at all, though some patients may exhibit gastrointestinal (GI) issues such as nausea, vomiting, anorexia, diaphoresis, and general malaise, typically within the initial 8 hours [9]. In *Stage II* (24–48 hours post-ingestion), GI symptoms may subside, but signs of hepatotoxicity, including elevated liver enzymes (AST and ALT), prothrombin time/International Normalized Ratio (INR), and bilirubin, start to appear, accompanied by right upper quadrant abdominal pain and tenderness, even though some patients may remain asymptomatic with a normal physical exam [10, 11]. *Stage III* (48–96 hours post-ingestion) represents the peak of hepatotoxicity, marked by severe hepatic dysfunction, which can manifest as coagulopathy, elevated hepatic enzyme levels, acidosis, hypoglycemia, jaundice, renal failure, anuria, cerebral edema, and coma [12]. Deaths from hepatic failure typically occur within 3–5 days of ingestion [13]. *Stage IV* (4–14 days post-ingestion) denotes the recovery phase, where liver function gradually returns to normal if the patient survives the acute phase [14].

5. Investigations

Paracetamol toxicity can result in life-threatening complications such as acute liver failure, metabolic imbalances, and multi-organ dysfunction. A suite of laboratory tests is vital for evaluating the extent of toxicity, informing treatment strategies, and predicting outcomes.

5.1 Serum acetaminophen concentration

The first step is to obtain a level at 4 hours post-ingestion or as soon as possible thereafter. Then, use the revised Rumack-Matthew nomogram for interpretation in acute ingestions, as shown in **Figure 2**.

The Revised Rumack-Matthew nomogram should only be applied after an acute acetaminophen ingestion. A serum acetaminophen concentration should be measured between 4 and 24 hours post-ingestion to ensure the peak level is captured. This concentration should then be plotted against the time of ingestion to assess the risk of toxicity and determine the necessity for treatment. If the plotted point falls on or above the treatment line, acetylcysteine therapy is recommended due to the potential for hepatotoxicity. For points on or above the high-risk line, many experts suggest administering a higher dose of acetylcysteine. The nomogram is not suitable when the ingestion history is unreliable or unknown, if ingestion occurred more than 24 hours before presentation, or in cases of repeated supratherapeutic oral ingestions or iatrogenic intravenous overdose. Refer to UpToDate for guidance on managing these

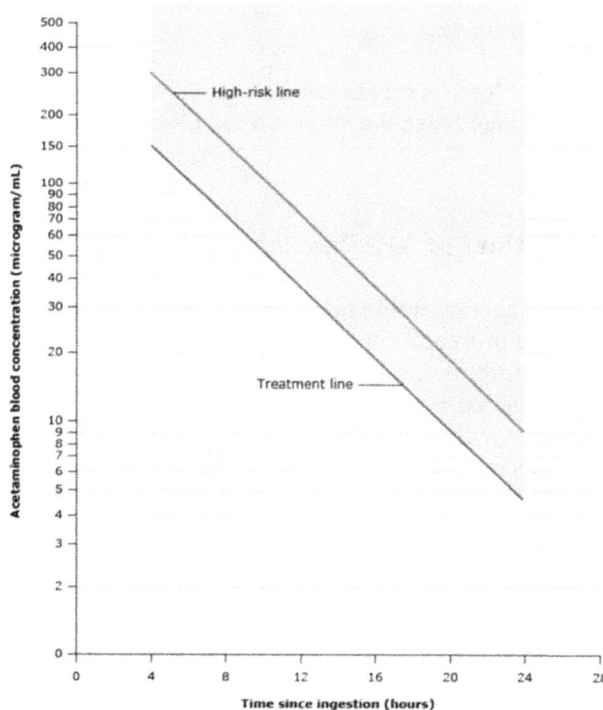

Figure 2.
Revised Rumack-Matthew nomogram.

situations and on when to repeat serum concentration measurements, particularly if an extended-release formulation was ingested or if there was co-ingestion with opioids or anticholinergics.

Not applicable for concentrations obtained before 4 hours, chronic, or repeated supratherapeutic ingestions [15, 16].

5.2 The Complete Blood Count (CBC) detects hematological changes secondary to liver impairment or systemic complications. For example, thrombocytopenia may signal advanced hepatic injury or coagulopathy, while leukocytosis could reflect systemic inflammation or infection.

Urea and electrolytes assess renal health, which may deteriorate due to dehydration, hypotension, or direct nephrotoxic effects of paracetamol. Imbalances such as hypokalemia or elevated creatinine often necessitate prompt correction to mitigate worsening renal function.

The Coagulation Profile, particularly prothrombin time (PT) and International Normalized Ratio (INR), is pivotal for gauging hepatic synthetic capacity. An elevated INR (>1.5) is a hallmark of liver dysfunction and a key prognostic marker in the King's College Criteria, used to evaluate the need for liver transplantation in acute liver failure.

Venous Blood Gas (VBG) analysis identifies acid-base disturbances, such as anion gap metabolic acidosis, which may arise from lactate accumulation due to hepatic necrosis or poor tissue perfusion. Severe acidosis or hyperlactatemia correlates with higher mortality and guides interventions like N-acetylcysteine (NAC) adjustments or critical care support.

Liver Function Tests (LFTs) remain central to diagnosing hepatocyte injury. Aspartate Aminotransferase (AST) levels rise rapidly within hours of overdose, reflecting acute cellular damage. However, AST's elevation lacks prognostic utility, as peak values do not predict survival or transplant eligibility. Instead, trends in INR, creatinine, and clinical signs (e.g., encephalopathy) are more reliable for outcome prediction [17, 18].

Also, several prognostic markers help predict outcomes in severe toxicity cases. Prothrombin time/INR remains a key determinant of liver function deterioration. Serum Bicarbonate or Blood pH provides insights into acid-base balance, where metabolic acidosis suggests severe toxicity. Serum Lactate is another crucial marker, with elevated levels indicating impaired tissue perfusion and mitochondrial dysfunction, often correlating with worse outcomes. Lastly, renal function tests help detect acute kidney injury, which can complicate severe cases of paracetamol overdose [3, 19].

Together, these tests aid in diagnosing paracetamol toxicity, monitoring disease progression, and guiding treatment decisions, including the need for N-acetylcysteine therapy or consideration for liver transplantation in critical cases.

6. Treatments approach

6.1 Airway and ventilation support

Maintaining a patent airway and ensuring adequate oxygenation are foundational in managing critically ill patients, particularly those with altered mental status due to hepatic encephalopathy, metabolic acidosis, or sepsis. Supplemental oxygen is administered initially via nasal cannula (2–6 L/min) or a non-rebreather mask (10–15 L/min) to target an SpO_2 ≥94%. Early intubation and mechanical ventilation are warranted in patients with a Glasgow Coma Scale (GCS) <8, refractory hypoxemia, or severe acidosis (pH <7.2), as these conditions pose a high risk of aspiration and respiratory failure. Lung-protective ventilation strategies, such as limiting tidal volumes to 6–8 mL/kg ideal body weight, are prioritized in cases complicated by acute respiratory distress syndrome (ARDS) to minimize further lung injury. Continuous monitoring via pulse oximetry and serial blood gas analysis (arterial or venous) guides adjustments in oxygenation and ventilation, while clinical assessments for encephalopathy (e.g., asterixis, confusion) ensure timely intervention for neurological decline [20].

6.2 Management of vomiting

Nausea and vomiting are addressed promptly to prevent complications such as aspiration, electrolyte imbalances, and delayed treatment adherence. Ondansetron (4–8 mg IV/oral), a serotonin receptor antagonist, is first-line due to its efficacy and safety in hepatic impairment, as it undergoes minimal hepatic metabolism. Metoclopramide (5–10 mg IV) is an alternative but is avoided in patients with bowel obstruction or Parkinson's disease due to extrapyramidal side effects. Refractory cases may benefit from adjuncts like dexamethasone (4–8 mg IV), particularly in chemotherapy-induced nausea or elevated intracranial pressure. Underlying contributors, such as hypokalemia or hyponatremia, must be corrected concurrently. In severe liver dysfunction, domperidone is avoided due to its reliance on hepatic metabolism, underscoring the importance of tailoring antiemetics to the patient's organ function [21].

6.3 Supportive care for organ failure

Hepatic and renal failure require meticulous supportive care to mitigate progression and complications. For hepatic encephalopathy, lactulose (30–45 mL orally or via nasogastric tube hourly until bowel movements occur) reduces ammonia absorption, with rifaximin (550 mg twice daily) added for recurrent episodes. Hypoglycemia, common in liver failure due to impaired gluconeogenesis, is managed with 10% dextrose infusions, avoiding concentrated solutions to prevent thrombophlebitis. Coagulopathy is addressed with vitamin K (10 mg IV) in malnutrition-related cases, while fresh frozen plasma (15–20 mL/kg) is reserved for active bleeding or pre-procedural stabilization. Renal failure necessitates careful fluid resuscitation with balanced crystalloids, avoidance of nephrotoxins (e.g., NSAIDs), and early nephrology consultation for dialysis in refractory acidosis (pH <7.1), hyperkalemia (>6.5 mmol/L), or uremic symptoms. Daily monitoring of electrolytes, creatinine, and fluid balance is critical to guide interventions [22, 23].

6.4 Gastrointestinal decontamination

In toxin ingestion (e.g., paracetamol overdose), the pre-ostomy intragastric pressure action is an efficient method of chemical decontamination. Activated charcoal (1 g/kg, max 50–100 g) is given within 1–2 hours after ingestion if the patient is awake and can protect their own airway. It strongly binds remaining toxins and plays a role in aiding antidotes such as N-acetylcysteine (NAC) for paracetamol toxicity. Gastric lavage or induced emesis are not usually attempted due to low efficacy beyond the first hour and high aspiration risk. The exceptions are whole-bowel irrigation with polyethylene glycol for sustained-release drug ingestions or body packers. Decontamination efforts should be made after ensuring the airway, and antidotes such as NAC are initiated immediately in suspected paracetamol overdoses, even before serum levels confirm toxicity, to prevent irreversible liver damage [24, 25].

6.5 N-Acetylcysteine (NAC) administration

N-acetylcysteine (NAC) is the preferred antidote for paracetamol (acetaminophen) poisoning, playing a critical role in preventing hepatotoxicity and acute liver failure. Its effectiveness is highly time-dependent, with early administration—ideally within the first 8 hours post-ingestion—significantly reducing the risk of liver injury [26]. Beyond this window, NAC can still provide benefits, particularly in cases of established toxicity, by replenishing glutathione stores and mitigating oxidative stress.

NAC is available in both oral and intravenous formulations, with specific dosing regimens tailored to each route of administration [27]. The intravenous form is preferred in patients with severe toxicity, altered mental status, or significant vomiting, whereas the oral formulation remains an option when intravenous access is not feasible. Regardless of the route, proper dosing and adherence to treatment protocols are crucial for optimal patient outcomes.

In cases of acute acetaminophen (APAP) toxicity, NAC initiation is based on the Revised Rumack-Matthew nomogram, which plots serum APAP levels against time since ingestion. If a patient's APAP concentration meets or exceeds the treatment threshold, NAC should be administered promptly to prevent hepatocellular damage [15].

For chronic overdoses, NAC is considered in patients who have exceeded safe daily limits, typically more than 4 g/day in adults or 120 mg/kg/day in children. High-risk individuals, such as those with chronic alcoholism, preexisting liver disease, or elevated liver enzymes, warrant particular attention, as they may develop toxicity at lower doses. In such cases, NAC administration can help prevent further hepatic injury and improve patient outcomes [28].

6.5.1 Dosing regimens

The dosing regimen for N-acetylcysteine (NAC) varies depending on the route of administration, with both intravenous and oral formulations available. The choice of route depends on the severity of toxicity, patient condition, and the presence of contraindications such as vomiting or altered mental status.

The intravenous NAC regimen (21-hour protocol) is delivered in three sequential infusions. The loading dose consists of 150 mg/kg administered over 60 minutes in 200 mL of 5% dextrose. This is followed by a second infusion of 50 mg/kg in 500 mL of 5% dextrose over the next 4 hours. The third infusion then provides 100 mg/kg in 1000 mL of 5% dextrose over 16 hours, bringing the total dose to 300 mg/kg over 21 hours. Upon completion of the protocol, liver function tests (LFTs), INR, and serum acetaminophen (APAP) levels should be reassessed. If APAP levels remain above 10 mcg/mL, AST/ALT exceeds 100 IU/L, or INR is greater than 1.5, NAC should be continued or restarted at the third infusion dose until laboratory parameters normalize [28].

For patients receiving oral NAC, the regimen consists of a loading dose of 140 mg/kg, followed by a maintenance dose of 70 mg/kg every 4 hours for 72 hours, totaling 17 doses. The cumulative NAC dose for this regimen reaches 1330 mg/kg over the full treatment

duration. While oral NAC is an effective alternative, its use is often limited by gastrointestinal intolerance, particularly in patients experiencing nausea or vomiting.

Both intravenous and oral NAC regimens are effective in preventing hepatic
injury when administered appropriately. However, timely initiation and continuous
monitoring of liver function and coagulation parameters remain critical to ensuring
successful treatment outcomes.

6.5.2 Anaphylactoid reactions

Anaphylactoid reactions are a well-recognized adverse effect of intravenous (IV)
N-acetylcysteine (NAC), occurring in approximately 5–30% of patients, particularly
during the initial loading dose infusion [29]. Unlike true anaphylaxis, these reactions are non-IgE-mediated and result from direct histamine release from mast cells
and basophils rather than immune system sensitization. Symptoms typically appear
within minutes to an hour of administration and can range from mild skin reactions
to more significant respiratory or cardiovascular effects.

The most common clinical manifestations include urticaria, pruritus, and
flushing, often accompanied by mild wheezing or dyspnea, particularly in individuals with asthma or reactive airway disease. Some patients may also experience
mild hypotension, though severe cardiovascular instability is rare. Risk factors for
anaphylactoid reactions include higher infusion rates, a history of atopy or asthma,
and female sex, which has been associated with a slightly increased likelihood of
adverse reactions.

Management of anaphylactoid reactions is primarily supportive, with the first step
being slowing or temporarily stopping the NAC infusion. In many cases, reducing
the infusion rate is sufficient for symptom resolution. For patients with urticaria and
flushing, H1-antihistamines such as diphenhydramine or promethazine are effective, and adding an H2-antihistamine like ranitidine may provide additional relief.
If bronchospasm occurs, treatment with inhaled beta-agonists such as salbutamol
may be necessary, particularly in asthmatic patients. Severe reactions with significant
hypotension are extremely rare but may require IV fluids, and in exceptional cases,
epinephrine may be considered.

Importantly, experiencing an anaphylactoid reaction does not mean that NAC
therapy should be discontinued. Once symptoms resolve, NAC can typically be
restarted at a slower infusion rate without recurrence of adverse effects. In rare
instances where IV administration is not tolerated, oral NAC may be considered as an
alternative. While anaphylactoid reactions to NAC can be concerning, they are generally mild, transient, and manageable with appropriate interventions, ensuring that
patients continue to receive the hepatoprotective benefits of NAC [29].

6.6 Acute single ingestion

The timing of the presentation is critical in determining the management
approach. For patients presenting between 4 and 8 hours post-ingestion, serum APAP
levels should be measured and plotted on the Revised Rumack-Matthew nomogram
to assess toxicity risk. If the APAP concentration is at or above 150 mg/L at 4 hours,
intravenous (IV) N-acetylcysteine (NAC) should be initiated to prevent hepatotoxicity. For patients presenting more than 8 hours post-ingestion, NAC should be started
immediately while awaiting APAP levels, as delayed treatment increases the risk of
liver injury [28].

6.7 Repeated supratherapeutic ingestion

In patients who have taken excessive doses of APAP over time, prompt laboratory assessment is necessary. Serum APAP and liver enzyme levels (AST/ALT) should be obtained as soon as possible. If APAP levels exceed 10 mg/L or if AST/ALT are elevated, IV NAC should be initiated without delay to minimize liver damage [28].

6.8 Extended-release APAP ingestion

Standard single-dose nomogram assessments may be insufficient due to prolonged drug absorption. APAP levels should be obtained at least 4 hours post-ingestion and then repeated after another 4 hours if the initial measurement falls below the treatment threshold on the nomogram. This ensures that delayed peaks in APAP concentration are identified and treated appropriately, reducing the risk of underestimating toxicity [28].

6.9 Fulminant hepatic failure

Intravenous N-acetylcysteine (NAC) plays a crucial role in improving survival, even when administered late in the course of toxicity. Unlike in early APAP poisoning, where NAC functions primarily as a glutathione precursor to detoxify N-acetyl-p-benzoquinone imine (NAPQI), in FHF, NAC is believed to exert additional hepato-protective and systemic benefits. These include reducing oxidative stress, improving microcirculation, and enhancing mitochondrial function, all of which support hepatic recovery in critically ill patients [28].

NAC should be continued until either liver function recovers or further intervention, such as liver transplantation, is warranted. Recovery is assessed based on clinical stability, improving hepatic biomarkers (AST, ALT, INR, bilirubin), and normalization of metabolic parameters. If progressive hepatic encephalopathy, worsening coagulopathy (INR >3.0), acidosis, or multi-organ failure develop despite NAC therapy, urgent evaluation for liver transplantation should be initiated. Early NAC administration remains the most effective strategy for preventing FHF, but even in late-stage toxicity, it provides significant survival benefits and should not be withheld unless contraindicated [28].

IV NAC improves survival and should continue until recovery or further intervention, such as liver transplantation, is warranted [28].

7. Follow-up

Any patient who develops gastrointestinal symptoms, abdominal pain, or jaundice after discharge should promptly return to the healthcare facility for evaluation. Patients with normal liver function tests following treatment with N-acetylcysteine (NAC) can resume therapeutic paracetamol (APAP). If acetylcysteine therapy is discontinued upon a toxicologist's advice and liver function tests show improvement but have not yet returned to baseline or normal values, it is expected that liver function will normalize within two weeks. During this period, patients are advised not to use paracetamol as a treatment for any condition. Once liver function normalizes, therapeutic paracetamol can be resumed, with the discontinuation of NAC guided by the toxicologist's recommendation [28].

8. Monitoring and prognosis

Effective management of acetaminophen (APAP) toxicity requires regular monitoring of key biochemical and clinical parameters to assess the patient's response to treatment and detect early signs of deterioration. Liver function tests (LFTs), including AST, ALT, bilirubin, and INR, should be monitored frequently to evaluate the extent of hepatic injury and the progression of liver dysfunction. Renal function (serum creatinine, blood urea nitrogen) and electrolyte levels should also be assessed, as acute kidney injury (AKI) can occur due to hepatorenal syndrome or direct nephrotoxicity associated with severe APAP overdose. Additionally, coagulation profiles (prothrombin time/INR) must be closely monitored, as worsening coagulopathy indicates declining hepatic synthetic function and may signal impending liver failure [30].

Among laboratory markers, elevated blood lactate levels have emerged as an early predictor of poor outcomes in paracetamol-induced acute liver failure. High lactate levels, particularly >3.5 mmol/L despite adequate fluid resuscitation, reflect impaired hepatic metabolism, mitochondrial dysfunction, and systemic hypoperfusion, all of which are associated with a higher risk of mortality and the need for liver transplantation [20]. Serial lactate measurements can aid in risk stratification, helping clinicians identify patients who may require intensified supportive care or urgent referral for liver transplantation. Regular and comprehensive monitoring ensures timely intervention, optimizing patient outcomes in APAP toxicity cases.

9. Conclusion

Acetaminophen (APAP) is a widely used medication due to its efficacy as an antipyretic and analgesic. However, it is also a leading cause of acute liver failure, primarily due to unintentional overdoses from various sources, including multiple medications containing APAP. Understanding the metabolism of APAP and its potential for toxicity is crucial for timely diagnosis and effective treatment of overdose cases. The management of APAP overdose involves a multi-faceted approach, including stabilization, decontamination, and the administration of N-acetylcysteine (NAC), the specific antidote. Early intervention is critical in preventing severe hepatotoxicity and ensuring patient recovery. By recognizing the signs and stages of APAP toxicity and applying appropriate therapeutic measures, healthcare professionals can significantly reduce the morbidity and mortality associated with this common yet preventable condition.

Acknowledgements

The completion of this chapter would not have been possible without the support and guidance of Sheik. Mohamed Hasan and my lovely wife Saja Mousa, their dedication and overwhelming attitude toward helping me is responsible for completing the chapter. The encouragement and insightful feedback were instrumental in accomplishing this task. The author acknowledges the use of free ChatGPT for language polishing and grammar refinement of the manuscript.

Author details

Mutwakil Elbidairi
Hamad Medical Corporation, Pharmacy Department, Doha, Qatar

*Address all correspondence to: melbidairi@hamad.qa;
motwkil_elbidairy@hotmail.com

IntechOpen

References

[1] Larson AM, Polson J, Fontana RJ, et al. Acetaminophen-induced acute liver failure: Results of a United States multicenter. Prospective Study. Hepatology. 2005;**42**:1364-1372

[2] Annual report of the American Association of Poison Control Centers Toxic Exposure Surveillance System. 2006. Available from: http://www.aapcc.org/archive/Annual%20Reports/06Report/2006%20Annual%20Report%20Final.pdf [Accessed: September 1, 2008]

[3] UpToDate. Uptodate.com. 2024. Available from: https://www.uptodate.com/contents/acetaminophen-paracetamol-poisoning-management-in-adults-andchildren?search=paracetamol%20poisoning&source=search_result&selectedTitle=1%7E103&usage_type=default&display_rank=1

[4] Graham G, Kieran FS. Mechanism of action of paracetamol. American Journal of Therapeutics. 2005;**12**:46-55

[5] Prescott LF. Absorption of paracetamol. In: Prescott LF, editor. Paracetamol (Acetaminophen). A Critical Bibliographic Review. London: Taylor & Francis; 1996. pp. 33-59

[6] Miller RP, Roberts RJ, Fischer LJ. Acetaminophen elimination kinetics in neonates, children and adults. Clinical Pharmacology and Therapeutics. 1976;**19**:676-684

[7] Mitchell JR, Jollow DJ, Potter WZ, et al. Acetaminophen-induced hepatic necrosis. I. Role of drug metabolism. The Journal of Pharmacology and Experimental Therapeutics. 1973;**187**:211-217

[8] FDA. Available from: http://www.fda.gov/ohrms/dockets/ac/02/briefing/Image1415.gif [Accessed: June 22, 2009]

[9] Prescott LF. Paracetamol: Past, present, and future. American Journal of Therapeutics. 2000;**7**(2):143-147

[10] Rumack BH, Matthew H. Acetaminophen poisoning and toxicity. Pediatrics. 1975;**55**(6):871-876

[11] Larson AM, Polson J, Fontana RJ, Davern TJ, Lalani E, Hynan LS, et al. Acetaminophen-induced acute liver failure: Results of a United States multicenter, prospective study. Hepatology. 2005;**42**(6):1364-1372

[12] Lee WM. Acetaminophen (APAP) hepatotoxicity—Isn't it time for APAP to go away? Journal of Hepatology. 2017;**67**(6):1324-1331

[13] Whitcomb DC, Block GD. Association of acetaminophen hepatotoxicity with fasting and ethanol use. Journal of the American Medical Association. 1994;**272**(23):1845-1850

[14] Makin AJ, Williams R. Acetaminophen-induced hepatotoxicity: Predisposing factors and treatments. Advances in Internal Medicine. 1997;**42**:453-483

[15] Dart RC, Mullins ME, Matoushek T, Ruha AM, Burns MM, Simone K, et al. Management of acetaminophen poisoning in the US and Canada: A consensus statement. JAMA Network Open. 2023;**6**(8):e2327739. Available from: https://jamanetwork.com/journals/jamanetworkopen/fullarticle/2808062

[16] Farrell SE. Acetaminophen Toxicity Clinical Presentation: History, Physical

Examination [Internet]. Medscape. com. Medscape; 2024 [cited 2025 Apr 11]. Available from: https://emedicine. medscape.com/article/820200-clinical?utm_source=chatgpt. com&form=fpf

[17] Agrawal S, Khazaeni B. Acetaminophen toxicity [Internet]. In: National Library of Medicine. StatPearls Publishing; 2023. Available from: https://www.ncbi.nlm.nih.gov/books/ NBK441917/

[18] Omalley G. Acetaminophen Poisoning [Internet]. Merck Manuals Professional Edition. Merck Manuals; 2018. Available from: https://www. merckmanuals.com/professional/ injuries-poisoning/poisoning/ acetaminophen-poisoning

[19] Dart RC, Mullins ME, Matoushek T, Ruha AM, Burns MM, Simone K, et al. Management of acetaminophen poisoning in the US and Canada: A consensus statement. JAMA Network Open [Internet]. 8 Aug 2023;**6**(8):e2327739. Available from: https://jamanetwork.com/journals/ jamanetworkopen/fullarticle/2808062

[20] Harrison PM, Wendon JA, Gimson AES, et al. Improvement by acetylcysteine of hemodynamics and oxygen transport in fulminant hepatic failure. The New England Journal of Medicine. 1991;**324**(26):1852-1857

[21] Rumack-Matthew H. Acetaminophen poisoning and toxicity. Pediatrics. 1975;**55**(6):871

[22] Lee WM et al. Intravenous N-acetylcysteine improves transplant-free survival in early-stage non-acetaminophen acute liver failure. Gastroenterology. 2009;**137**(3):856-864

[23] Keays R, Harrison PM, Wendon JA, et al. Intravenous acetylcysteine in

paracetamol-induced fulminant hepatic failure: A prospective controlled trial. BMJ. 1991;**303**(6809):1026-1029

[24] Hendrickson RG, Bizovi KE. Acetaminophen. In: Goldfrank's Toxicologic Emergencies. 8th ed. New York, NY: McGraw-Hill; 2006

[25] O'Grady JG, Alexander GJM, Hayllar KM, Williams R. Early indicators of prognosis in fulminant hepatic failure. Gastroenterology. 1989;**97**(2):439-445

[26] Smilkstein MJ, Knapp GL, Kulig KW, et al. Efficacy of oral N-acetylcysteine in the treatment of acetaminophen overdose. The New England Journal of Medicine. 1988;**319**(24):1557-1562

[27] Bernal W et al. Blood lactate as an early predictor outcome in paracetamol-induced acute liver failure: A cohort study. Lancet. 2002;**359**(9306):558-563

[28] Fisher ES, Curry SC. Chapter ten - Evaluation and treatment of acetaminophen toxicity [Internet]. In: Ramachandran A, Jaeschke H, editors. Vol. 85. ScienceDirect. Academic Press; 2019. pp. 263-272. Available from: https://www.sciencedirect.com/science/ article/abs/pii/S1054358918300504

[29] Abdrabbo M. TOXCard: Acetaminophen Toxicity and Management. emDOCs.net - Emergency Medicine Education. 2018. Available from: https://www.emdocs.net/ toxcard-acetaminophen-toxicity-and-management/

[30] Schmidt LE, Dalhoff K. Serum phosphate is an early predictor of outcome in severe acetaminophen-induced hepatotoxicity. Hepatology. 2002;**36**(3):659-665

Chapter 4

A New Insight into Mechanism of Mushroom Poisoning

Sumitra Debnath

Abstract

In many parts of the world, particularly in hilly areas with humid weather, mushrooms are a common edible fungus. The majority of mushroom poisoning deaths worldwide are caused by amatoxin. Around the world, 56,679 species of macrofungi, or mushrooms, have been recognized. People have traditionally considered mushrooms to be a delicacy and a valuable addition to their diets. Liver and renal failure are among the many organ dysfunctions brought on by amatoxin, along with gastrointestinal issues. The causes of mushroom poisoning, species causes poisoning, its symptoms, some conventional and contemporary treatment options, and preventative measures will all be covered in my chapter.

Keywords: edible mushroom, poisonous mushroom, mechanism of toxicity, treatment, precautions

1. Introduction

Mushrooms are the sporocarp of fungi and comprise a source of sustenance. In specific cultures and nations, a variety of wild or field mushroom species are regarded as exquisiteness. However, it can be challenging to distinguish between "edible" and "deadly" mushrooms, as many of them can be harmful if consumed. In addition, some "edible" species can prove toxic to some humans in certain circumstances, which may not be predictable. In our nation, eating naturally cultivated mushrooms is a rather prevalent habit, particularly among rural residents. Hundreds of patients are admitted to hospitals each year with mushroom poisoning, and many of them pass away due to the complications. More than 5000 kinds of fungi are known to produce mushrooms, which are their visible sporocarp. However, just around 100 of these are toxic and are responsible for the majority of mushroom poisoning incidents. The clinical manifestation caused by poisonous chemicals present in mushrooms is called "mycetismus," or mushroom poisoning. Because cool, wet evenings promote the growth of mushrooms, spring and fall are the most common seasons for mushroom poisoning. Mushroom poisoning remains a health problem that causes morbidity and mortality in many countries. It is unknown how many people die each year from eating mushrooms worldwide, although it is estimated to be at least.

100 deaths annually. This number is likely underestimated, given that between 50 and 100 deaths occur annually in Europe alone [1].

Farmers who gather mushrooms mistakenly identify dangerous (*Amanita phalloides*) and edible mushrooms due to their similar shapes and colors, which causes poisoning all over the world. While established poisoning syndromes are being reported outside of their previously identified zones of incidence, the majority of mushroom species have undisclosed toxicology, and new poisoning syndromes are persistently skyrocketing. The secondary metabolites that are present are the result of particular metabolic pathways within the fungal cell. *Amanita phalloides*, also known as the "death cap," is responsible for the majority of fatal poisonings worldwide. Other harmful mushroom species include *Amanita verna*, *Amanita virosa*, Gyromitra, Gallerina, and Lepiota species, all of which contain the powerful cytotoxin amatoxin. Even a small amount of one deadly kind of mushroom may be enough to kill a person. Teenagers purposefully ingest "magic" mushrooms because of their psychedelic properties. It frequently takes the expertise of a group of scientists, including doctors, botanists, and mycologists, to accurately identify the toxin. The clinical manifestations of mushroom poisoning depend mainly on the type of mushroom involved (the degree of toxic species), amount ingested (obvious), age (symptoms in children are more fatal compared to an adult due to their having low body weight), time of onset of symptoms (very toxic mushroom poisoning cases usually have delayed onset of symptoms which are very severe with hepatic, renal, hemolytic, and CNS involvement), geographic distribution, as well as premorbid hepatic and renal condition.

2. Morphological features of mushrooms

- Primordia, which are nodules or pinheads that are less than two millimeters in diameter and are usually found on or close to the substrate's surface, are the precursors of mushrooms.

- Mushrooms are filamentous fungi with many cells.

- It is created within the mycelium, the bundle of thread-like hyphae that make up the fungus.

- They typically grow on rotten logs, tree trunks, soil rich in organic matter, dung cakes, decomposing organic matter, etc.

- Mushrooms belong to the kingdom Fungi or Mycota.

- They are achlorophyllous (lack chlorophyll) and hence cannot prepare their own food.

- Mushrooms rely on dead, decaying organic matter for sustenance because they are achlorophyllous, meaning they lack chlorophyll and cannot produce their own food.

- There are two types of mushrooms: edible and non-edible (toxic or poisonous).

- The layer of microscopic spore-bearing cells covering the gill surface is called a hymenium.

- The hymenium covers the teeth of spine fungus and coral branches, or it lines the inside surfaces of the tubes of boletes and polypores in non-gilled mushrooms.

- Spores grow inside tiny, sac-like cells called asci, which are found in the Ascomycota. Each ascus normally contains eight spores.

- The Discomycetes, which include the brain, sponge, cup, and several club-like fungi, produce an exposed layer of asci, such as inside morel pits or on the inside surfaces of cup fungi.

- The asci grow inside the tiny, flask-shaped perithecia produced by the Pyrenomycetes, which are dark-colored fungi that thrive on a variety of substrates such as soil, manure, leaf litter, and rotting wood.

- Four spores often form on the tips of sterigmata, which are slender projections that emerge from club-shaped cells known as basidia in basidiomycetes. The Gasteromycetes' fertile part, known as a gleba, can turn slimy like the stinkhorns or powdery like the puffballs.

- Paraphyses are thread-like sterile cells that are scattered throughout the asci. Similar structures known as cystidia are frequently found in the Basidiomycota's hymenium. There are many different kinds of cystidia, and determining their size, shape, and existence is frequently used to confirm a mushroom's identity.

3. Species and its clinical toxicities

Only perhaps 50–100 of the 10,000 types of mushrooms that grow worldwide are known to be hazardous. One mushroom (50 g) can kill an average adult (LD 50) at a rate of 0.2–0.75 mg/kg body weight. When making a differential diagnosis for any episode of acute gastroenteritis, it is important to consider the possibility of mushroom poisoning throughout the spring and fall, when mild temperatures and moist circumstances promote the growth of mushrooms. The vast majority of poisonings are not fatal, but the majority of fatal poisonings are caused by the *Amanita phalloides* mushroom. Although the majority of mushroom poisoning incidents are unintentional, there is evidence that they can occasionally be purposeful. Most Poison Center calls are about possible ingestions by young children, particularly toddlers grazing in the backyard. The majority of adult "poisonees" are amateur mushroom collectors who eat the mushrooms they harvest. Most illnesses are self-limited gastrointestinal reactions, and a significant but unknown percentage of those who are afflicted never seek medical help. It is important to note that some reactions are unique and involve fungi that are often consumed and that people who eat them accept. However, mistaken wild fungi are responsible for nearly all severe poisonings. Tragic errors are especially prone to occur when *Agaricus bisporus* (death cap) is involved. Death caps can be mistaken for edible Volvariella species, including the paddy straw mushroom, which is utilized in Southeast Asian cooking, by some of these pickers. Unfamiliarity with US species also causes poisoning among other immigrant groups, including those from Eastern Europe, Mexico, and Central America. Classification of Mushrooms is explained in **Figure 1** and **Table 1**.

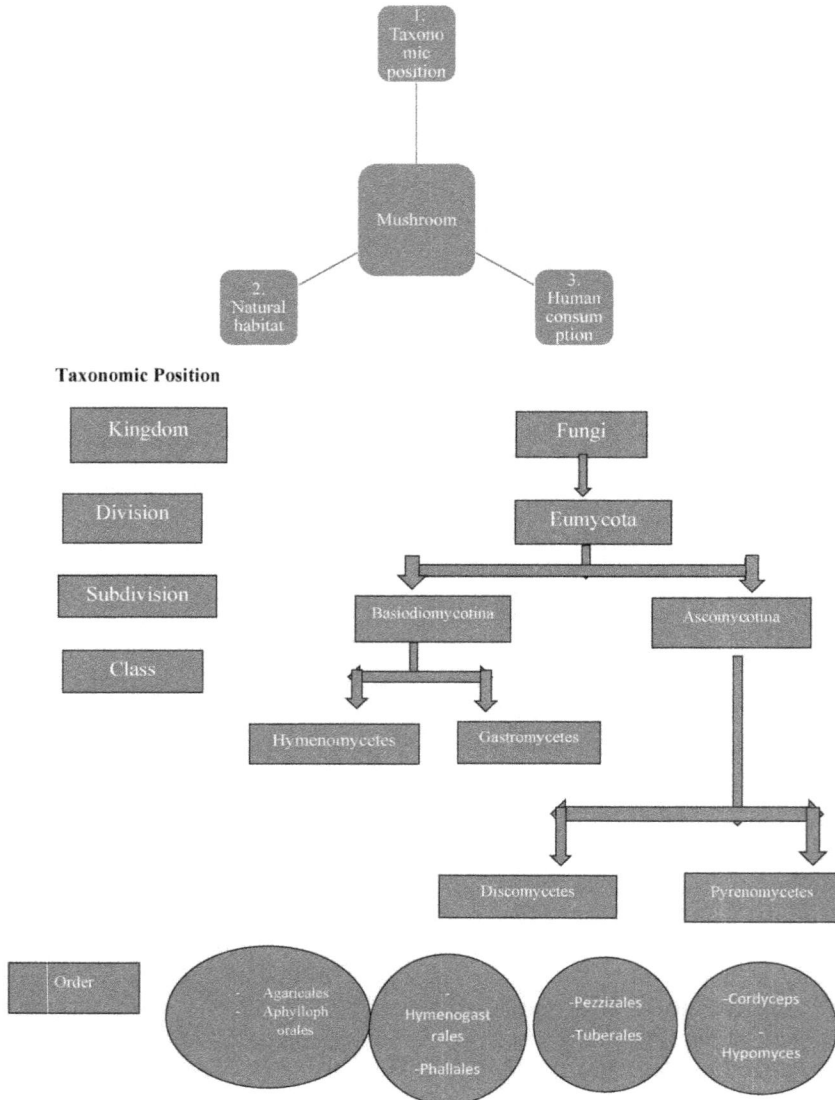

Figure 1.
Classification of mushroom.

Inhabiting media	Terminology	Saprophytic	Parasitic/Symbiotic
Humus	Humicolous/Folicolous	*Marasmius* spp. *Volvariella* spp. *Polyporous* spp	Boletus Lactarius, Tricholoma spp. (S)
Wood	Lignicolous	*Agrocybe* spp. *Pleurotus* spp. Lentinus edodes	*Armillaria mellea Cyttaria* spp. (P)

Table 1.
Natural habitat.

In ecology, a particular organism lives in a particular natural environment and gives the best result.

4. Human consumption

4.1 Edible mushroom

Edibility may be defined by criteria that include the absence of poisonous effects on human and desirable taste and aroma [2].

1. Paddy straw mushroom (*Volvariella volvacea*)

2. Oyster mushroom (*Pleurotus ostreatus*)

3. Button mushroom (*Agaricus bisporus*)

4. Milky mushroom (*Calocybe indica*)

5. Shiitake mushroom (*Lentinula spp.*)

6. Jew's ear mushroom (*Auricularia spp.*)

4.2 Non-edible mushroom

Some mushrooms are not edible because of their growing environment or the way they smell or taste, i.e., quite unpleasant [2].

4.3 Poisonous mushroom

Poisonous mushrooms are called toadstools.

1. *Amanita phalloides*

2. *Amanita virosa*

3. *Cortinarius rubellus*

4. *Amanita pantherine*

5. *Amanita muscaria*

6. *Chlorophyllum molybdites*

7. *Psilocybe semilanceata*

4.3.1 Edible mushroom

4.3.1.1 Volvariella volvacea

The edible mushroom species *Volvariella volvacea*, also referred to as paddy straw mushroom or straw mushroom, is widely used in Asian cooking and is grown throughout East and South East Asia. In areas where they are grown, they are usually sold fresh, while in other place, they are more commonly found dried or canned. The Paddy Straw Mushroom (*Volvariella volvacea*), also referred to as the Chinese mushroom or straw mushroom, is a member of the Basidiomycetes family Pluteaceae. It is a tropical and subtropical edible fungus that was originally grown in China in 1822. At first, this fungus was referred to as "Nanhua mushroom," after the Nanhua Temple in China's Northern Guangdong Province. Paddy straw mushroom is also known as "warm mushroom" as it grows at a relatively high temperature. On a fresh weight basis, it is composed of approximately 90% water, 30–43% crude protein, 1–6% fat, 12–48% carbohydrates, 4–10% crude fiber, and 5.13% ash, based on the information currently available. The fruiting body's fat content increases to up to 5% as it reaches a fully grown stage [3].

4.3.1.2 Pleurotus ostreatus

A common edible mushroom is *Pleurotus ostreatus*, also known as the oyster mushroom, oyster fungus, hiratake, or pearl oyster mushroom. Although it may be grown on straw and other medium, it is one of the most popular wild mushrooms. It has been said that the mushroom has a moderate flavor and a faint anise-like smell. The oyster mushroom is best harvested when it is young because as it ages, its meat gets tough and its flavor is bitter and disagreeable. Oyster mushrooms have long been an essential part of traditional cuisine as a rich source of nutrients and folk medicine because of its many health advantages. Beta-glucan, which is found in oyster mushrooms, supports heart health by lowering blood cholesterol levels. Oyster mushrooms contain lovastatin, which helps manage cholesterol levels in the blood. Of all the farmed mushrooms, oyster mushrooms have the highest niacin content. More than half of your daily requirement of vitamin B3, which supports the proper operation of your muscles and nervous system, may be found in just 100 grams of oyster mushrooms. The growth of breast and colon cancer cells is inhibited by oyster mushrooms. They prevent the spread of cancer cells to other parts of the body. Oyster mushrooms' glycoprotein naturally strengthens the body's anti-cancer defenses. Oyster mushrooms are rich in polysaccharides, which have been shown in numerous studies to help stop the formation of tumors.

4.3.1.3 Agaricus bisporus

The cultivated mushroom, or *Agaricus bisporus*, is a basidiomycete mushroom that is native to grasslands in North America and Eurasia. One of the most popular and extensively consumed mushrooms worldwide, it is grown in over 70 countries. When it is juvenile, it has two color states: brown and white. Each of these states has a variety of names, and when it is mature, it has additional names such as button, champignon de Paris, portobello, chestnut, and portabellini. The use of A. bisporus in numerous traditional medicines has a long history. Extracts from *A. bisporus* and/or its bioactive compounds are being used more and more around the world as antioxidants, anti-cancer, and anti-inflammatory agents to treat a variety of human illnesses, including cancer, diabetes mellitus, bacterial and fungal infections, immune system disorders, and coronary heart disease. Although there have been relatively few direct intervention trials of mushroom consumption in humans, those that have been completed to date indicate that mushrooms and their extracts are generally well-tolerated with few, if any, side effects [4].

4.3.1.4 Calocybe indica

The milky white mushroom, or *Calocybe indica*, is a type of edible mushroom that is indigenous to India. The robust, all-white mushrooms grow on roadside verges and in fields following summer rains. Traditionally consumed in West Bengal, it is now commercially farmed in a number of Indian states as well as other tropical nations. The nutritional value of milky mushrooms is similar to that of other types of mushrooms. On a dry weight basis, the mature fruit body of *C. indica* has the highest protein content (17.2%), while the juvenile pin heads have the lowest protein content (15.2%), along with 4.1% fat, 3.4% crude fiber, and 64.26% carbohydrates. Approximately 7.43% ash, 2.9% starch, and 4% soluble sugars are present in mature fruit bodies. Alanine, aspartic acid, glutamine, glutamic acid, glycine hydroxyl proline, histidine, lysine, threonine, tryrosine, valine, arginine, and proline are the twelve amino acids found in the fruit body. Glycine is the most abundant amino acid (10.8 g/100 g protein). Furthermore, it contains all of the mineral salts—potassium, sodium, phosphorus, iron, and calcium—that the human body needs. It is ideal for those who suffer from constipation and hyperacidity because of its high fiber content and alkaline ash. According to Ragul [5], the dry weight percentage of chitosan derived from *C. indica* sporophores varied between 2.5 and 2.9%. According to reports, the beta-glycans found in the dietary fibers of mushrooms have antimutagenic, anti-cancer, and anti-tumor properties that stimulate the immune system.

4.3.1.5 Lentinula spp.

A small genus of agarics that live on wood is called Lentinula. Shiitake, or Xiang-gu in Chinese, is the Japanese name for the nutrient-dense edible and medicinal fungus species *Lentinula edodes* (Berk.) Singer. With an annual production of about 7 billion kg, shiitake mushrooms (*Lentinula edodes* L.) are thought to be the most widely grown mushrooms in the world, accounting for 22% of the global mushroom supply. Proteins, dietary fibers, essential amino acids, and numerous vitamins, including B1, B2, B12, C, D, and E, can be found in these mushrooms. They also contain a variety of medicinal compounds, such as lipids, polysaccharides, sterols, and terpenoids, which have anti-tumor, anti-viral, anti-hypertensive, and immune-modulatory properties. There are a number of uses for *Lentinula edodes*, such as the production of bioethanol, the nematicidal activity of its spent mushroom compost against nematodes like *Panagrellus* spp., the improvement of wheat utilization in poultry production by xylanase enzymes, bioindicators for soil pollution, medicinal qualities, biotechnology because they prevent chronic diseases, particularly diabetes and hypercholesterolemia, as a source of bio-elements, and the biocontrol of plant diseases like strawberry leaf spot, which is caused by *Xanthomonas fragariae*. Numerous morphologically unique mycoviruses or virus-like particles are present in this mushroom. Because of its low production costs, stability, adaptability to incorporate functional ingredients, ease of transportation, and positive reception, this mushroom's nutritional complexity could be turned into a functional food (similar to functional bars). The shiitake mushroom can be eaten as dried fruiting bodies that smell like toast or garlic, or as fresh fruiting bodies in a variety of culinary meals.

4.3.1.6 Auricularia spp.

Auricularia are usually ear-shaped and gelatinous, it has a smooth, wrinkled, or veined underside and an upper surface that is noticeably hirsute to mildly downy.

Wood is the foundation for all species. Common names for Auricularia auricula-judae include wood ear, jelly ear, and, more traditionally, Jew's ear. The B complex vitamins and numerous other bioactive substances, including polysaccharides that enhance heart function, are abundant in wood ear mushrooms. A study that was published in "Mycobiology" claims that it lowers the atherogenic index by 40% and helps control cholesterol levels. This metric is used to forecast the likelihood of heart disease and artery plaque accumulation. A study that was published in "Thrombosis and Hemostasis" examined the amount of adenosine found in wood ear mushrooms. Adenosine is a chemical byproduct of the body's cellular metabolism that affects heart health, blood pressure, and blood coagulation. In addition to other unknown substances that support Wood Ear's capacity to prevent platelet aggregation and blood clotting, researchers found that one gram of the dried mushroom contains 154 mcg of adenosine. It has also been discovered that the polysaccharides in wood ear mushrooms affect platelet aggregation and coagulation, which may help prevent thrombosis. It has been discovered that mannose, glucose, glucuronic acid, and xylose prevent platelet aggregation and blood clotting. In addition to preventing heart attacks, strokes, and arterial damage that can result in heart disease, this can help to improve circulation. The wood ear mushroom is incredibly rich in antioxidants. Its antioxidant properties have been shown to help stop the onset of degenerative diseases, including dementia and Alzheimer's. According to a 2013 study in the "International Journal of Medicinal Mushrooms," eating raw or cooked wood ear mushrooms may shield the brain from these two crippling illnesses. Furthermore, cooking the mushrooms can increase their antioxidant activity, according to a 2019 study published in the "Journal of Food Science and Technology." Wood Ear Mushroom-derived β-glucan exopolysaccharides have the ability to stimulate the immune system. They increase the activity of phagocytes, which are immune cells that defend the body by consuming germs, dead or dying cells, and dangerous foreign objects. Additionally, they contain a lot of dietary fiber—roughly 71% of it is insoluble fiber. Until the last segment of the large intestine, insoluble fiber is not broken down. According to recent research, bacteria in the colon can break down this fiber to create a lot of short-chain fatty acids (SCFAs), primarily butyric, propionic, and acetic acid. These SCFAs help maintain digestive health and reduce the risk of colon issues by supplying energy to the cells lining the intestinal wall. For thousands of years, wood ear mushrooms have been a mainstay of traditional Chinese medicine. When fresh, this type of mushroom has a firm, gelatinous, elastic texture. Its exterior surface is bright reddish brown with a tint of purple, and it is frequently covered in tiny, gray, downy hairs. It also, predictably, looks a lot like an ear. The Wood Ear Mushroom is also often used in Asian cooking. Its mild woody flavor and crisp texture make it a great addition to salads, soups, and stir fries.

4.3.2 Poisonous mushrooms

4.3.2.1 Amanita phalloides

One of the many dangerous basidiomycete fungi and mushrooms in the genus Amanita is *Amanita phalloides*, also referred to as the death cap. Among all known mushrooms, *Amanita phalloides* is the most toxic. According to estimates, an adult human can be killed by the toxin in as little as half a mushroom. It is also the most deadly fungus in the world, accounting for 90% of all fatalities caused by mushrooms annually. Cooking does not lessen the harmful effects of amatoxin, the class of toxins present in these mushrooms, because they are thermostable and resist changes brought on by heat. Amatoxins, phallotoxins, and virotoxins are the three types of cyclic peptide toxins found in *Amanita phalloides*. A minimum of nine distinct molecules, including α-amanitin, β-amanitin, γ-amanitin, ε-amanitin, amanin, amaninamide, amanullin, amanullinic acid, and proamanullin, combine to create amatoxin, a bicyclic octapeptide. A sulfur atom replaces the tryptophan residue at position 2 of the indole ring in all categories of poisons. Amatoxins are extremely deadly and can kill a person in 2–8 days, but virotoxins and phallotoxins are less toxic but act more quickly, killing a person in 2–5 hours. *A. phalloides* poisoning has a high death rate because it contains amatoxins, which are powerful toxins. Since the liver and kidneys are the most metabolically active organs, α-amanitin is typically the cause of damage following ingestion. The chemical structure and bioactivity of virotoxins are thought to be similar to those of phallotoxin since they are thought to be formed from the same precursor. After consumption, neither virotoxins nor phallotoxins are significantly harmful. In light of the recent warm weather and heavy rainfall, members of the Bay Area Mycological Society informed staff at the California Poison Control System (CPCS) on November 28, 2016, of an exceptionally big *A. phalloides* bloom in the wider San Francisco Bay Area. The first human *A. phalloides* poisoning of the season was reported to CPCS 5 days later. Thirteen more cases of hepatotoxicity from consumption of A. phalloides were reported to CPCS within the next 2 weeks. Prior to this outbreak, CPCS had only been notified of a small number of annual instances of mushroom poisoning.

4.3.2.2 Amanita virosa

The European destroying angel is the common name for the fungus species *Amanita virosa*, which is a member of the Agariomycetes class. In late summer and fall, it can be found in woodlands, especially with beech and chestnut, but it can also be found with pine, spruce, and fir. The fruit bodies, or basidiocarps, are pure white, agaricoid (mushroom-shaped), and have a volva at the base that resembles a sack and a ring on the stem. The fruit bodies of *Amanita virosa* contain both amatoxins and phallotoxins, and the fruit has a pure white appearance, like a veil of angels, with smoother roots than *A. verna*. Because of its deadly nature, it has been dubbed "The destroying angel." As with other Amanita mushrooms, it has a sweet smell and taste, and the center of the fruit turns yellow or brown as it matures. *Amanita virosa* is highly toxic and has been the cause of severe mushroom poisonings; an adult human can be killed by eating just one cap, and a delay in symptoms may make treatment more difficult. The white spores of *A. virosa* have a diameter of 8–10 mm and a length-to-width ratio of less than 1.25. The red and white *A. muscaria*, commonly referred to as "fly agaric," is one of the most exquisite and common species of Amanita. Monocyclic peptides made up of at least five distinct substances are known as virotoxins. They may have similar precursor routes because of their similar biological activity and structure to phallotoxins. Phalloidin and amanitin are the two primary poisons of *A. phalloides*.

Phalloidin (MW of 900 Da) was found in *A. phalloides* in 1937 [5], and phallotoxins were initially found in *A. virosa* in 1974. Although its presence in *A. virosa* was still up for debate, amanitin—mostly alpha-amanitin, with a molecular weight of roughly 900 Da—was discovered in this species in 1966. It is interesting to note that *A. phalloides* and other Amanita species generate γ-amanitin, while *A. virosa* may create amaninamide. According to most research conducted to date, *A. virosa* includes two primary amatoxins, beta-amanitin and alpha-amanitin, as well as two phallotoxins, phalloidin and phallacidin. Amaninamide and alpha-amanitin, but not beta-amanitin, were discovered in *A. virosa* in a study conducted by some researchers. The findings published by Yocum and Simons after the chemical analysis of *A. virosa* mushrooms gathered from several US regions corroborated these findings. Virotoxins are monocyclic peptides that share similarities with phallotoxins in their biological function. While some investigations revealed virotoxins in both A. subpallidorosea and *A. virosa* species, other articles claimed that virotoxins were only found in *A. virosa*. Based on phylogenetic study, *A. virosa* and *A. subpallidorosea* are grouped together. Furthermore, prior research indicates that the properties of toxin cyclopeptide align with phylogenetic molecular linkages. The majority of the virotoxins were discovered in mushrooms that were gathered from North America and Europe. The toxovirin that was isolated from *A. virosa* exhibits strong oxidase activity for particular amino acids but no mono- or diamino-oxidase activity. The impact of toxovirin on L-amino acids is twice as great as that of DL-racemic combinations. The toxophallin that was isolated from *A. phalloides* shares structural and chemical similarities with this toxin. In 2016, the monocyclic peptide viroidin cyclopeptide was discovered in *A. virosa* for the first time. Other Amanita species, such as *A. bisporigera* and *A. verna*, have the ability to create toxic peptides (amatoxin, phallotoxins, and virotoxin), just like *A. phalloides* and *A. virosa*. Instead of seven amino acids, amatoxins contain eight. Once more, two side chains are joined by a sulfur atom; the hydroxyl group (highlighted) is crucial for toxicity.

4.3.2.3 Cortinarius rubellus

Cortinarius rubellus, also known as the deadly webcap, is a type of fungus that is native to temperate to subalpine woods in high latitudes in North America and Eurasia. Its features include a pale yellow flesh, adnexed to sinuate gills that are yellow-brown to rusty-brown, a dry yellow-brown to red-brown stem that is club shaped or wider in the center, with yellowish veil bands; a domed to umbonate to peaked non-hygrophanous to slightly hygrophanous, dry orange-brown to reddish-brown cap that is wooly fibrillose to fibrillose squamulose; radish to indistinct odor and taste; habitat of conifers; basidiospores are ornamented, subglobose to broadly elliptical or elliptical, with significant shape variation [6]. It belongs to a class of very deadly organisms called Orellani. *Cortinarius rubellus* contains the powerful myco-toxin orellanine. In Finland, the risk of poisoning was initially identified in 1972 following four occurrences, two of which led to irreversible renal failure. Three visitors to the Inverness region were poisoned in 1979 because they thought it was chanterelle. Kidney transplants are required for two of the three. Nine of the twenty-two individuals who were poisoned in Sweden between 1979 and 1993 needed a kidney transplant after developing end-stage renal failure (ESRF). They confused the mushroom with a number of culinary species, including chanterelles, Hygrophorus species, and *Craterellus tubaeformis*. The funnel-shaped cap and ridges on the underside of the cap, rather than gills, are characteristics that set the edible *Craterellus tubaeformis* apart. It was consumed in 1996 by an Austrian who was searching for miracle mushrooms. The so-called "Orellanus syndrome," which is characterized by a loss of kidney function, can appear up to 3 weeks [2–6] prior to renal failure. It frequently results in severe kidney damage, dialysis, or even death from *C. orellanus* or *C. rubellus* intoxication. However, as far as we are aware, no published investigation has documented orellanine in blood samples following intoxication with *C. rubellus* or *C. orellanus*. According to Wieland and Faulstich [6], "Orellanine can be detected after a relatively long period following poisoning by performing a simple thin layer chromatography technique using small quantities of renal biopsy material." When C. orellanus or *C. rubellus* intoxicates a patient, the presence of orellanine in the kidney is described using thin layer chromatography (TLC). There were no toxins in the urine or blood tests. Another paper states that the existence of orellanine was indirectly proven "by assaying orellanine in the plasma and two renal biopsies of patient after specific photo-decomposition into a non-toxic metabolite called orel-line" [6]. Inhibiting the oxidative defense and producing oxygen radicals, orellanine functions by downregulating most antioxidative enzymes.

4.3.2.4 Amanita pantherine

Amanita pantherine is a toxic and psychedelic fungus that grows throughout Eurasia. It is also referred to as the panther cap, false blusher, and panther amanita because of its resemblance to the actual blusher (*Amanita rubescens*). "The fatality rate [for *A. pantherine*] is probably less than 1%, but reports are still inadequate" [7, 8]; yet, this mushroom can be lethal if consumed in high numbers (five or more caps). It is dark brown, hazel-brown, or pale ochraceous brown, with many easily removable warts that range in color from pure white to squalid cream. It is also minutely verruculose and floccose. It has a short striate border and becomes viscid when moist. When wounded, the white flesh remains unchanged. *A. pantherine* is distinguished by its elliptical, inamyloid spores and the collar-like roll of volval tissue at the top of the basal bulb, in addition to its brownish cap with white warts. The epithet "false blusher" comes from the fact that, in contrast to panther, *Amanita rubescens* cap does not turn red or pink ("blush") when the flesh is injured. This is a crucial characteristic that sets the two species apart. Although *A. pantherine* is poisonous, humans may not die from eating it fresh. It can result in vomiting, diarrhea, and hyperhidrosis, all of which can induce extreme dehydration. Ibotenic acid and muscimol, two psychoactive substances found in *A. pantherine*, can produce hallucinations, synaesthesia, euphoria, dysphoria, and retrograde amnesia, among other effects. The effects of ibotenic acid and muscimol are more like those of a Z drug, such as Ambien at large dosages, than they are of a traditional psychedelic, such as psilocybin. Because A. *pantherine* is significantly more strong and less identifiable than its much more recognizable sibling *A.muscaria*, it is utilized as an entheogen far less frequently. Since ancient times, people have been aware of the psychedelic qualities of *A. muscaria* (L. ex Fr.) Hooker (fly agaric) and *A. pantherine* (panther cap). Mysticism is associated with the use of the fly agaric and the panther hat. From July to October, *A. pantherine* is frequently found in Poland's coniferous forests. The panther cap grows in both coniferous and deciduous woodlands, particularly birch and beech. *A. pantherine's* crown is 5–10 cm in diameter, gray or gray brown, gray yellow, pale when old, and contains tiny, pure white flakes. This species has occasionally been confused with the edible *A. rubescens* in unintentional poisoning instances in Poland.

4.3.2.5 Amanita muscaria

Amanita muscaria (L.) Lam. is the most recognizable mushroom in contemporary popular culture because of its unusual red crown with white dots. Many languages use its vernacular names, fly agaric and fly amanita. In fact, it has been used for generations in European houses to trap flies by steeping them in a bowl of milk since it attracts and intoxicates them. Although this fungus is believed to be deadly, it has been eaten as food in a number of countries, including Mexico and Italy, when it is fresh. The water that contains the majority of the water-soluble poisonous chemicals is removed after boiling the mushroom in many traditional recipes. The mushroom is dried, immersed in brine for 12 weeks, and then washed several times before being eaten in Japan. However, this mushroom's popularity is neither new nor exclusive to cooking, as people have been consuming it for thousands of years; it has affected religious and spiritual beliefs, especially in Neolithic Siberian societies. A lot of tales, stories, and representations show how symbolic the fly agaric is to our collective imagination. *A. muscaria* is a fungus that belongs to the Amanitaceae family, the order Agaricales, and the division of the Basidiomycota. It typically grows in podzolic soils from deciduous and coniferous forests. In these acidic soil conditions, nitrogen is primarily found in its poorly mobile ammonium and organic forms, and bacterial rates of nitrogen mineralization of the leaf litter are low. *A. muscaria* plays a crucial role in the nitrogen uptake of plants in these environments through mycorrhizal symbiosis due to its high-affinity ammonium importer gene. These symptoms include intoxication, hallucinations, restlessness, elevated psychomotor drive, depression of the central nervous system, and gastrointestinal disturbance. The typical clinical course after consuming fly agaric includes cramps, tremor, ataxia, nausea, vomiting, diarrhea, and incoordination after 30 minutes. After 60 minutes, a changed mental state is observed, characterized by deteriorating senses, alternating between agitation and obtundation, and strange actions, such as confusion and depersonalization. Visual and auditory abnormalities are frequent types of hallucinations. Last but not least, the side symptoms imply fatigue followed by restful sleep. There is not a cure at the moment because the symptoms are both cholinergic and anticholinergic. After ingestion, supportive care for symptoms, the use of activated charcoal, and gastro-intestinal lavage are common therapies. On the other hand, fatalities are extremely uncommon, and it is quite improbable that consuming a cap will cause death. However, it was shown that the lethal dosage for an adult human would be 15 caps. In addition to its acute toxicity, the fungus can also be consumed as food during detoxi-fication, and the caps may store toxins. Therefore, regularly eating mushrooms that have been harvested in dangerous areas may result in chronic toxicity associated with extended exposure to heavy metals.

4.3.2.6 Chlorophyllum molybdites

The toxic mushroom *Chlorophyllum molybdites* (G. Mey) Massee, sometimes referred to as the "false parasol" or "green-spored parasol," is a member of the Agaricaceae family. This family includes the majority of "parasol" mushrooms, including a number of edible species. *Chlorophyllum molybdites* is said to be the most common cause of mushroom poisoning in the United States. This hazardous spe-cies is commonly mistaken for edible mushroom species like the shaggy parasols (*Chlorophyllum rhacodes, C. olivieri, and C. brunneum*) or the true parasol mushroom (*Macrolepiota procera*). *Chlorophyllum molybdites* are found in temperate and subtrop-ical climes across the planet, including in parks and lawns in eastern North America. Fruiting bodies usually appear after summer and fall precipitation. *Chlorophyllum molybdites* may be a prolific fruiter and frequently creates "fairy rings" in enormous circles and semi-circles on lawns. It has the ability to yield a lot of fruit. Even though *C. molybdites* is not as lethal as some other species, it is important to identify this common fungus because it is present in many disturbed environments, such as residential yards and agricultural fields. The gastrointestinal irritant toxin produced by *C. molybdites* can generate severe symptoms when ingested. All parts and stages of the mushroom contain the toxin; however, the cap has a higher concentration than the stem, gills, and spores. Lab testing shows that the poison can affect humans, dogs, mice, and chickens. One to two hours after consumption, symptoms such as nausea, vomiting, diarrhea, and loss of fluids and electrolytes may manifest. In more extreme situations, these symptoms can lead to hypotension and hypovolemic shock, a disease in which the body goes into shock due to blood or fluid loss. The intensity of these symptoms might vary from mild to severe. Symptoms may last 4 hours or up to 7 days, depending on the amount of toxin ingested and the severity of poisoning. The majority of patients recover in a day, but those who suffer from hypovolemic shock and dehydration take longer to recover. The reported differences in *C. molybdite* toxicity from case to case may be due to genetic variances among populations, the substrate the mushroom was growing on, the age of the mushroom, and the climate at harvest. Additionally, each person has a unique tolerance to the toxin due to differences in gastrointestinal pH and stomach pepsins. According to studies, the toxin is labile after 30 minutes of heating to 70°C (158°F) and is water soluble, indicating that cooked *C. molybdites* mushrooms are probably less hazardous than fresh ones. Young children and dogs are more susceptible to poisoning by this species than adults because they are smaller (i.e., have less body mass) and more likely to eat fresh mushrooms that grow in lawns. The simplest technique to identify mushroom poisoning in children and pets who show symptoms is to look for uneaten bits of the mushroom and, if possible, greenish spores in the vomit. There is currently no recognized treatment for *C. molybdite* toxicity. A hospital emergency room or other healthcare institution should be used to determine the severity of the poisoning.

4.3.2.7 Psilocybe semilanceata

Psilocybin mushrooms are often referred to as magic mushrooms or hallucinogenic mushrooms. Psilocybin mushrooms are a polyphyletic informal group of fungi that contain psilocybin, which when consumed transforms into psilocin. Members of the genus Psilocybe, notably *P. cyanescens*, *P. semilanceata*, and *P. azurescens,* are the most powerful species; however, psilocybin has also been isolated from about a dozen additional genera, including Panaeolus (which includes Psilocybe, Conocybe, Gymnopilus, and Pholiotina). Psilocybin mushrooms are utilized as recreational drugs, among other cultural uses. They are most likely represented in pre-colombian sculptures and glyphs found in the Americas, while they may also be observed in stone age rock art in Africa and Europe. The makeup of magic mushrooms differs from species to species and from genus to genus. Its main ingredient, psilocybin, is transformed into psilocin to cause intoxicating effects. In addition to psilocin, other substances that may be present and alter the effects of magic mushrooms include norpsilocin, baeocystin, norbaeocystin, and aeruginascin. Psilocybin and psilocin are what give psilocybin mushrooms their effects. The liver undergoes a process known as dephosphorylation when psilocybin is consumed. The resultant substance, psilocin, is what gives psychedelic effects. Users' tolerance is temporarily increased by psilocybin and psilocin, which makes it harder to abuse them because the more frequently they are taken in a short period of time, the less potent the effects become. There is no evidence that psilocybin mushrooms can result in either psychological or physical reliance (addiction). After consumption, the psychedelic effects start to manifest about 20 minutes later and can continue for up to 6 hours. Physical side effects could include exhilaration, nausea, vomiting, tiredness, lack of coordination, and muscular weakness or relaxation. The effects of psychedelic mushrooms are subjective and can differ significantly from person to person, as is the case with many psychedelic substances. The duration of psilocybin-containing mushrooms' mind-altering effects varies from 3 to 8 hours, contingent on individual metabolism, preparation technique, and dosage. The "peak" is usually defined as the first 3–4 hours following ingestion, during which the user perceives more vivid images and reality distortions. Because psilocybin can change how time is perceived, the benefits may seem to stay considerably longer for the person. The "trip," or experience, is highly reliant on the environment, just like other psychedelics like LSD. It is common to experience humor, inattention, and muscle relaxation. Because psychedelics intensify experiences, a person who goes into a trip feeling worried is likely to experience increased anxiety during the trip. For many users, taking the mushrooms alongside friends or others who are accustomed to "tripping" is preferred. Hallucinations and a loss of the ability to distinguish between reality and fiction are among the psychological effects of psilocybin use. Psychosis and panic attacks can also happen, especially if a person consumes a lot of the drug. The "LD50" or median lethal dose of psilocybin is 280 mg/kg. A person who is anxious before a trip is likely to feel more anxious while on it, since psychedelics heighten experiences. Taking the mushrooms with friends or other people who are used to "tripping" is preferred by many users. The psychological effects of psilocybin use include hallucinations and a loss of the ability to discriminate between reality and fantasy. Additionally, if a person uses the medicine excessively, they may experience panic episodes and psychosis. Significantly high psilocin levels can overstimulate the brain's 5HT2A receptors, resulting in acute Serotonin Syndrome, which is a more plausible concern than a fatal overdose. According to a 2015 study, mice given 200 mg/kg of psilocin experienced acute serotonin overdose symptoms. The majority of patients referred to critical care are discharged with relatively mild treatment, making neurotoxicity-induced fatal outcomes rare in cases of psilocybin mushroom abuse. However, excessive psilocybin mushroom use can result in deadly events associated with emotional discomfort and trip-induced insanity. A 27-year-old man who had succumbed to hypothermia was discovered dead in an irrigation canal in 2003. Two psilocybin mushroom growing pots were discovered in his bedroom; however, no toxicological report was filed. Research on psilocybin mushrooms' potential to cure drug dependence, anxiety, and mood disorders was limited in the United States until the early twenty-first century, in part because of the Controlled Substance Act's prohibitions. For psilocybin research in depressive disorders, the Food and Drug Administration (FDA) awarded Breakthrough Therapy Designation in 2018–2019.

5. Mechanism of toxicity of mushroom

α-Amanitin toxicity is dependent on RNA polymerase II inhibition, which in turn inhibits the transcription process. Other harmful processes, primarily the production of reactive oxygen species, have also been hypothesized. Furthermore, α-amanitin may potentially function as a co-adjuvant to trigger apoptosis in conjunction with endogenous cytokines such as tumor necrosis factor-α to induce apoptosis [9]. Apoptosis is also a major factor in the severe hepatic damage caused by amanitin, since a concentration of amanitin in liver cells results in apoptosis that is dependent on p53 and caspase3.

The concentration needed for promotion of p53 was related with the concentration needed to decrease mRNA production, supposing a relationship between these two effects. The decrease in mRNA concentration leads to inhibition of protein synthesis, which ultimately results in cell death. By forming p53 complexes with protective protein (Bcl-xL and Bcl-2), moving p53 from the cytoplasm to the mitochondria, and releasing cytochrome c into the cytoplasmic space, oxidative stress can also contribute to amanitin toxicity by altering the permeability of the mitochondrial membrane. According to Letschert et al. [8], high hepatic amanitin concentration causes the production of free radicals and other reactive species, as well as an increase in superoxide dismutase (SOD) and malondialdehyde products and decrease in catalase concentration. According to Bonnet et al. [10], lipid peroxidation also contributes significantly to the widespread necrosis and severe liver damage, and phenoxyl free radicals may be implicated in the production of ROS. Its psychedelic effects are known to be caused by two main compounds: Muscimol and Ibotenic acid. Ibotenic acid is a neurotoxin that functions as a pro-drug to muscimol; following decarboxylation, about 10–20% of it transforms into muscimol. When consumed, just 53 mg of muscimol is needed to elicit psychoactive effects; 93 mg of muscimol causes severe intoxication, including vomiting. Effects were detectable in human volunteers around 1 hour after 7.5–10 mg of muscimol, or 50–90 mg of ibotenic acid, was consumed. These effects linger for 3 to 4 hours, and in certain patients, the residual effects can last for 10–24 hours. It was found that consuming 20 mg of ibotenic acid and 5 mg of muscimol, lassitude, and sleepiness. Muscarine, ibotenic acid, muscimol, and muscazone are the primary toxins found in *A. muscaria*. Vanadium (an organometallic compound called amavadine) and other hazardous metals are known to be effectively bio-accumulated by the mushroom. Ibotenic acid also contains tricholomic acid, stizolobinic acid, and stizollobic acid as derivatives. L-Dopa oxidation products, which are known to have anticholinergic effects, are connected to these three molecules. Muscimol and ibotenic acid share structural similarities. While ibotenic acid is an agonist of NMDA glutamate receptor interactions that cause the hallucinogenic effects seen during intoxication, muscimol, which shares structural similarities with GABA, is a strong agonist of the GABAA receptor. Ibotenic acid is a colorless, crystalline chemical that dissolves in water. It is also known as (S)-2-Amino-2-(3-hydroxyisoxazol-5-yl) acetic acid. It is converted to an equivalent amount of muscimol that crosses the blood-brain barrier by decarboxylation in the stomach, liver, and brain. Within an hour of exposure, both compounds can be found in urine. In contrast to muscimol, ibotenic acid is far more harmful, resulting in seizures and lesions in particular parts of the brain that resemble Alzheimer's disease, for which it is employed in animal test. GABA transaminase, the enzyme that breaks down GABAA and the GABAA uptake systems are not affected by the non-selective GABAA receptor agonist muscimol, which also reaches the brain through peripheral injection. Muscimol is partial agonist of GABAc receptors and non-selective agonist of GABAA receptor and it activates both pre- and post-synaptic receptors. It is said to be a strong agonist at post-synaptic receptors in the mammalian central nervous system that are strychnine-insensitive and bicuculline-sensitive.

For instance, muscimol (3 mg/kg, i.p.) causes the brain's serotonin levels to rise while catecholamine levels fall. The substance primarily binds to GABAA receptors in the thalamus, the hippocampus, the caudate nucleus, and the putamen in the forebrain. This causes the receptor linked to the chloride ion channel to open, which in turn inhibits neuronal activity. According to a mouse knockout study, a certain population of GABAA receptors that may have subunit 6 and lack subunit 1 were necessary for the high-affinity binding of muscimol in forebrain regions such as the caudate putamen, thalamus, and hippocampus. The panther cap's effects do not take long to manifest. Cooking does not significantly reduce toxicity. Human clinical signs have been documented 30 minutes to 2 hours following *A. pantherine* consumption. One cap is usually enough to produce psychoactive effects. Tropanic alkaloids are absent from the "mycoatropinic" poisoning symptoms caused by fly agaric and panther cap. CNS depression with lethargy, gradual obtundation, and ataxia is typically the initial symptom.

6. Pathophysiology

The clinical presentation differs depending on the species of mushroom and toxin ingested.

Acute gastroenteritis: The most common cause of acute gastroenteritis is one of the many "backyard mushrooms" such as *Chlorophyllum molybdites*. The great majority of reported poisonings are caused by symptoms of nausea, vomiting, cramping in the abdomen, and occasionally diarrhea. Usually, it appears in 1 to 3 hours.

6.1 Hallucinations

Caused by psilocybin and species that contain it, such as *Psilocybe*, *Conocybe*, *Gymnopilus*, and *Panaeolus*. These substances bind to 5-hydroxytryptamine (5-HT) subtype receptors as agonists or partial agonists. Although they may grow naturally in warm, humid regions, these are cultivated and misused for recreational reasons. Either dried mushrooms or fresh mushroom caps can be consumed. Depending on the dosage, altered sensorium and euphoria remain for 4–12 hours after ingestion and start 30 minutes to 2 hours later.

6.2 Cholinergic toxicity

Muscarine-containing species from a variety of taxa, including Clitocybe and Inocybe, are the cause of cholinergic poisoning. Small quantities of muscarine are present in Amanita muscari, but usually not enough to provide a cholinergic appearance. Abdominal cramps, diaphoresis, lacrimation, salivation, bronchospasm, bronchorrhea, and bradycardia are among cholinergic symptoms that often manifest within 30 minutes. In contrast to other cholinergic poisoning causes like pesticides, the duration is dose-dependent but usually brief.

6.3 Disulfiram-like reaction

Brought on by species that contain coprine, such as Coprinus atramentarius, frequently referred to as "inky cap," The metabolites of the toxin block aldehyde dehydrogenase, which results in flushing, tachycardia, headache, nausea, vomiting, and, in rare instances, hypotension. This only occurs if coprine-containing mushrooms are eaten hours or days after consuming alcohol. The effects are lessened when alcohol and the toxin are consumed together because coprine's conversion to its toxic metabolites occurs more slowly.

6.4 Liver toxicity

The primary pathophysiological consequence of mushroom poisoning is hepatic failure. In Amanita species, amatoxin is the primary cause. They cause RNA polymerase II to malfunction, which results in cellular protein deficiencies. Three separate phases are characteristic of toxicity.

Usually, the gastrointestinal effects begin 6–12 hours after administration and then subside 24–36 hours later, during which time symptoms start to recover.

However, there can be laboratory evidence of hepatotoxicity during this stage. Massive centrilobular hepatic necrosis was discovered by hepatic histological analysis. Hepatitis can develop suddenly, leading to unconsciousness and liver failure. Massive necrosis and fatty degeneration are visible in hepatic cells. Because hepatic failure reduces the removal of clotting factors and the excretion of procoagulants from degenerated hepatic cells, it may result in disseminated intravascular coagulation. All of these things result in multiple organs. Hepatic damage worsens after 48 hours, resulting in liver failure and its aftereffects. In severe situations, liver transplantation may be necessary, or death may occur within a week.

6.5 Nephrotoxicity

Orellanine is a nephrotoxic substance produced by members of the Cortinarius genus. After consumption, renal symptoms could appear 1 to 2 weeks later. Acute tubular necrosis and renal shutdown are additional symptoms of Amanita phalloides poisoning. Additionally, renal tubular acidosis of the post-Fanconi type may develop. Acute gastroenteritis symptoms usually appear first, followed by kidney damage within 12 to 24 hours. With the right supportive care, the majority of patients recover completely, however, some will need hemodialysis.

6.6 Seizures

Seizures caused by gyromitrin, which is found in species of Gyromitra, Paxina, and Cyathipodia micropus, both of which are far less prevalent. Foragers may inadvertently ingest Gyromitra while searching for morel (*Morchella esculenta*). The metabolite responsible for the toxicity is monomethylhydrazine, which leads to pyridoxine (B6) and ultimately GABA depletion. Anticonvulsant drugs may therefore be unable to manage these seizures, requiring further treatment, such as pyridoxine.

6.7 Central nervous system

Ammonia buildup (a byproduct of protein catabolism) is brought on by hepatorenal insufficiency, since ammonia is converted to urea by the renal system and then eliminated by the kidney. This raises blood levels of ammonia, which can cross the blood-brain barrier and result in encephalopathy. According to Jander and Bischoff [11], the process ultimately results in the principal neurological manifestation linked to Amanita phalloides. Secondary neurologic symptoms result from liver and renal failure as well as a reduction in blood pressure.

6.8 Other manifestations

Numerous more clinical signs may arise due to the wide variety of mushrooms that might be consumed. Erythromelalgia (acromelic acid), dermatitis (shiitake mushrooms), rhabdomyolysis (Tricholoma equestre), methemoglobinemia, hemolysis (*Paxillus involutus*), migraines, vertigo, somnolence, palpitations, and dysrhythmias are a few of these.

7. Clinical signs of mushroom toxicity

1. The amatoxin is actively harming the cells of the liver and kidneys during the first phase, which lasts for 6 to 24 hours after eating. The patient typically does not complain of any symptoms at this point. This phase averages 10 hours.

2. The second stage: Individuals frequently get diarrhea during this time. According to Garcia et al. [12], diarrhea that starts within 8 hours is a sign of a poor prognosis. The second stage of poisoning is characterized by diarrhea, emesis, nausea, and cramping in the abdomen. Hyperpyrexia, palpitations, a drop in blood sugar, a drop in blood pressure, dehydration, and an acute electrolyte imbalance are some of the symptoms that might accompany these symptoms. This gastrointestinal stage is frequently accompanied by vomiting and bloody diarrhea. During this phase, liver and renal function tests are often within the normal range.

3. The third phase: a 24-hour period in which the patient looks to be recovering, despite kidneys and liver damage, which is proven by renal, hepatic function. Elevated Serum transaminases and lactic dehydrogenase, and jaundice will develop and become apparent [13]. If the patient is discharged without evaluation of liver and kidneys functions, this may lead to death.

4. The fourth phase: A significant rise in transaminase levels, coagulopathy, delirium, headache, hyperbilirubinemia, oliguria, uremia, hepatic encephalopathy, hepatorenal syndrome, and acute renal failure are the hallmarks of the fourth phase, also known as fulminant hepatitis or the hepatic failure stage. One to three weeks following consumption, there may be multiple organ failure, disseminated intravascular coagulation, convulsions, and even death. Rapid improvement in liver function tests and symptoms is a common characteristic of patients who will fully recover.

8. Diagnosis

- Muscarinic toxidrome is characterized by weakness, pinpoint pupils, cramping in the muscles, and noticeable respiratory symptoms.

- Sometimes RBC cholinesterase levels.

In patients with neuromuscular and respiratory signs, especially those who are at risk, the diagnosis is typically made based on the distinctive muscarinic toxidrome. Reversal or reduction of muscarinic symptoms with 1 mg of atropine (0.01 to 0.02 mg/kg in children) supports the diagnosis in cases where the results are unclear. If at all possible, the particular toxin should be determined. Numerous organophosphates have distinct smells, such as gasoline or garlic. The degree of poisoning is indicated by RBC cholinesterase activity, which some labs can quantify.

Although patient response is the main indicator of success, values can be used to track how well a treatment is working if it can be measured quickly.

9. Treatment of mushroom poisoning

9.1 Primary assessment and initial care

Activated charcoal and GASTRIC LAVAGE prevent amatoxin from being absorbed through the gastrointestinal tract, although this method works best when patients get to the emergency room soon after ingesting the toxin. This strategy loses effectiveness because the patient takes longer to get to the hospital because of the latent phase, which starts right after eating mushrooms and lasts for around 6 hours.

9.2 Many dosages of charcoal activation

When given shortly after intake, they may be useful in lowering gastrointestinal absorption following gastric lavage. However, the purpose of this approach was to stop the enterohepatic circulation of amatoxins when there was a delay in the delivery of activated charcoal.

9.3 Rehydration

Since vomiting and diarrhea brought on by amanita phalloides mushroom poisoning result in dehydration, sometimes severe dehydration causes a decrease in renal blood flow, which in turn causes renal insufficiency. Dehydration also raises the level of lactic acid and causes metabolic acidosis. In order to sustain and prevent irreversible hepatic failure, intravenous fluid delivery is crucial for correcting these metabolic anomalies.

9.4 Diuresis

Since amatoxin is eliminated through the kidneys, induced diuresis plays a significant part in enhancing toxin removal.

9.5 Hemodialysis and hemoperfusion

Hemodialysis and hemoperfusion have a positive impact when amatoxin enters the bloodstream and is seen in plasma, even though they have no bearing on the outcome. Nonetheless, other research indicates that it has a positive effect on patients' survival.

9.6 Plasmapheresis

Although plasmapheresis, the other detoxification method, is unable to remove a high enough concentration in relation to renal excretion, it can supply the albumin, immunoglobulins, coagulation factors, fibrinolytic proteins, and mineral salts that are necessary for the resuscitation of hepatic cells.

9.7 Antidotes

A. phalloides poisoning can benefit from the use of certain medications that increase the excretion of amatoxin, such as silymarin, benzylpenicillin, and N-acetylcysteine. However, there is no particular antidote for amatoxin.

9.8 Penicillin G or benzyl penicillin

Competition with amatoxin for binding sites on plasma proteins, particularly albumin, is how it works. By blocking OATP1B3 receptors, the second mechanism prevents hepatocytes from absorbing amatoxin. Gamma-aminobutyric acid (GABA) is synthesized by normal intestinal mucosa flora. Amatoxin induces the liver to degrade this substance, therefore, benzyl penicillin lowers the GABA level and prevents encephalopathy by killing the intestinal normal flora.

9.9 N-acetylcysteine (NAC)

As an amatoxin that induces oxidative stress, which in turn results in GSH depletion, NAC functions as a precursor to glutathione. Another antioxidant that helps reduce toxicity is ascorbic acid, which protects liver cells from harm and death caused by free radicals. Second, lipid peroxidation of cell membranes, oxidation of proteins and nucleic acids, and damage to all cell components are caused by reactive oxygen species. These events lead to glutathione depletion and cell death. NAC scavenges free radicals in a non-specific manner, preventing cell damage. NAC has been shown to increase non-transplant survival and be beneficial in grade I–II encephalopathy.

9.10 Cimetidine

Amatoxin is changed into the active form of toxic amatoxin, amanitin, by the cytochrome P450 enzyme. Cimetidine stops this harmful biotransformation by inhibiting this enzyme.

9.11 Silibinin

Extract of silymarin, a flavolignan obtained from the seeds of the milk thistle (Silibinin), can be beneficial when the mushroom eating has been ongoing for 2 days. It works by blocking OATP1B3 receptor systems, which stops intestinal and liver cells from absorbing amanitin.

By demonstrating a protective effect and lowering the mortality rate, it improves the prognosis.

Anticholinergic drugs like atropine or glycopyrrolate may be useful in treating cholinergic toxicity. Adults should take 0.5–1 mg of atropine intravenously; children should take 0.01 mg/kg. Pyridoxine (B6) should be given specifically to those who have refractory seizures as a result of consuming Gyromitra. Pyridoxine at a dose of 25 mg/kg IV can be used as a therapy or as a prophylactic to control seizures. Benzodiazepines might be a helpful addition [14, 15]. Those who have swallowed amatoxin should be especially aware of N-acetylcysteine (NAC), silibinin, and penicillin. Practitioners should use the local toxicology resource or poison control center while evaluating and managing patients.

10. Biological replacement therapy

10.1 Hemodialysis

Dialysis functions as an artificial renal system in medicine, removing waste products, excess fluid, and harmful compounds from the bloodstream. Only in cases where a patient has consumed a potentially fatal quantity of carbamazepine, dapsone, phenobarbital, quinine, or theophylline should multiple-dose activated charcoal be considered. Hemodialysis can alleviate the encephalopathy associated with amanitin poisoning, although it has no positive effect on mushroom toxicity.

10.2 Polymyxin B

It works by attaching itself to the amanitin binding site on RNAP II, preventing amanitin from binding to RNAP II and significantly reducing the harm that toxins cause to the liver and kidneys. Additionally, by lowering the death rate, it enhances the long-term prognosis.

10.3 Liver transplantation

Hepatic transplantation can save a patient with a poor prognosis and improve their condition if they arrive at the hospital late or are not treated appropriately, which can lead to fulminant liver failure.

10.4 Prognosis

Most mushroom ingestions that result in gastrointestinal symptoms will go away without any problems if the right supportive care is provided. One study found that 68% of patients who took Cortinarius had renal impairment, with 11% suffering from end-stage renal failure and 51% requiring hemodialysis. Twelve of the 90 patients in the cohort eventually had kidney transplants. After receiving supportive care and appropriate seizure control, the majority of patients who consume Gyromitra recover in less than a week. A 10% mortality rate was discovered in one study conducted in Eastern Europe. According to one research, 2% of patients with Amanita toxicity eventually needed a liver transplant. Mildly hepatotoxic patients typically recover. Although refractory bradycardia, shock, and death have been reported in cases of severe anticholinergic toxicity, patients with mild anticholinergic toxicity usually recover.

11. Improving healthcare team results

The symptoms of mushroom toxicity are diverse, necessitating an interdisciplinary approach to patient care. Physicians and nursing personnel need to be aware that, depending on the local environment, non-specific gastrointestinal symptoms may be related to the absorption of mushroom toxins. Treatment cannot be prompt and effective if this diagnosis is not on the differential. Since they will spend the most time at the patient's bedside assessing for any changes or decompensation, technicians and nurses play a critical role in their treatment. For many of these toxidromes, the patient may continue to worsen over the course of hours, even if the initial presentation may seem benign. For more information and suggestions, the medical staff should get in touch with the local poison control centers as soon as possible. The majority of information regarding management and treatment for certain mushroom poisonings comes from case reports, case studies, or expert opinion, just like with many other toxic ingestions and wilderness medicine (Level V). The majority of mushroom ingestions are treated with supportive care. Specialists in the domains of kidney, liver, and neurology should be consulted while managing these manifestations. N-acetylcysteine, pyridoxine, methylene blue, atropine, and glycopyrrolate are examples of antidotes that should be administered in accordance with toxicologist recommendations.

12. Patient education and deterrence

The majority of mushroom poisonings cause mild to severe gastrointestinal symptoms, such as diarrhea, vomiting, and nausea. Nevertheless, a number of aftereffects might result in organ failure and even death. Foragers, especially those who are new to the activity, need to be aware of the wide variety of mushroom species and their mimics. For amateur foragers, understanding the edible and hazardous fungus species in the area is essential. Evaluation is necessary for even minor nausea since it may be a sign of a serious illness.

13. Discussion

Young children who accidentally consume mushrooms, people who hunt for mushrooms in the wild, people who are trying to commit suicide or murder, and people seeking a hallucinogenic high are the four primary types of people who can become poisoned by mushrooms [16]. The mushrooms they gathered from the wild poisoned the patient. Based on when symptoms first appear, the numerous clinical syndromes of mushroom poisoning are divided into three categories: early (less than 6 hours), late (6–24 hours), and delayed (more than a day). Pantherine syndrome is categorized as an early-onset glutaminergic neurotoxic condition.

Humans have been known to experience clinical symptoms 30 minutes to 2 hours after ingesting *A. pantherine*, and these symptoms can persist for up to 12 hours [17, 18]. Muscle spasms, delirium, hallucinations, nausea, and profound sleep are all signs of pantherine syndrome. Additionally, there have been reports of mydriasis, hallucinations, ataxia, bradycardia, confusion, dizziness, fatigue, visual and aural sensitivities, and dry mouth. The last stage of poisoning is coma. Usually, just one mushroom cap is enough to produce psychoactive effects. This poisoning is mainly characterized by neurologic symptoms and dysfunctions of the central nervous system. Lethargy and hyperkinetic behavior, as well as delirium and obtundation, are possible symptoms. Adults rarely get seizures. In our instance, the primary symptoms were hallucinations and a reduction in consciousness that began around 30 minutes after the mushrooms were consumed. Neurotoxic isoxasoles, ibotenic acid, and muscimol are the active toxins in *A. pantherine* that cause poisoning symptoms. Muscimol stimulates GABA receptors, while isotelic acid stimulates NMDA receptors. The amount of poisons is unaffected by cooking. The patient consumed the sautéed mushrooms. Similar symptoms can also be caused by *A. muscaria*. Confusion, agitation, hallucinations, convulsions, slumber, coma, vomiting, and diarrhea are all possible side effects of both mushrooms. While *A. pantherine* has more inhibitory muscimol, *A. muscaria* has more excitatory ibotenic acid. As a result, poisoning with *A. muscaria* more frequently induces agitation and disorientation, while poisoning with *A. pantherine* more frequently results in coma [19]. The patient was placed in a coma. Instead of trying to identify the fungus, the patient's symptoms should be the primary guide for the supportive treatment. It is advised to use gastric lavage and activated charcoal to remove the mushroom from the digestive system. The symptoms are usually minimal and do not need to be treated further. They respond to standard treatment with benzodiazepines and other anticonvulsants if seizures do occur. Additionally, benzodiazepines should be given to treat delirium and agitation. Patients experiencing bradycardia symptoms should be the only ones prescribed atropine. Comas from severe poisonings may require intubation. For certain patients, intensive care is advised. In our instance, agitations were treated with benzodiazepines. Although *A. pantherine* poisoning is rarely fatal, the prognosis is usually favorable. After 24 hours, healing is usually almost total with no discernible aftereffects. In 15 hours, the patient recovered. In cases of repeated intake, severe neuronal and even brain damage may be expected. Two crucial components of treatment are education and prevention [20]. Recalling specifics about individual mushrooms is not as critical as remembering the toxidromes. Mushrooms come in thousands of species. For efficient maintenance, knowing the precise species of mushroom may be useful, although it is not necessary. Non-lethal mushrooms typically start to show symptoms within 6 hours, but since patients frequently consume multiple types of mushrooms, this does not necessarily mean that a potentially harmful species was also consumed. It can be useful for identification if any mushrooms are still present. The emergency physician assessed the remaining mushrooms that the patient had brought for diagnostic purposes, but regrettably, they were not submitted to a mycologist for confirmation and analysis. The diagnosis is aided by a history of mushroom consumption and the associated toxidrome, however, the symptoms might vary and are easily mistaken for benign clinical disorders like gastroenteritis. Due to the lack of a single, effective counteragent, severe amanitin-induced mushroom intoxication is still an open issue in clinical toxicology. Better outcomes from mushroom poisoning depend on early discovery and timely treatment.

14. Conclusion

Particularly among the Indian subcontinent's rural and tribal communities, mushroom poisoning is a serious issue. Nevertheless, the issue is underreported and mostly ignored. More research is required to fully comprehend the significance and severity of mycetism, particularly in the huge Indian subcontinent, as epidemiological studies on mushroom poisoning are insufficient worldwide. The ultimate goal of preventing and treating mushroom poisoning may be accomplished in collaboration with clinicians, funding agencies, mycologists, researchers, government and public officials, and non-governmental organizations. Such initiatives can also draw the attention of government policymakers and health authorities. To confirm the diagnosis of mushroom toxicity, researchers and physicians should be encouraged to carry out comprehensive studies to comprehend the poisons and their pathophysiology. It takes money and appropriate facilities to create novel antidotes for mushroom poisons. Since there are now no known particular antidotes, "prevention is better than a cure" should be taken into consideration in order to lower the mortality and morbidity associated with mycetism. The incidence of mushroom poisoning will be further decreased by creating a database of deadly mushrooms particular to a given area, raising public awareness of suspicious mushroom gathering, and improving infrastructure at primary rural health centers. The present study was conducted on the basis of information available on Wikipedia and the scientific papers, and further investigations are needed to find out more about mushroom toxicities.

Conflict of interest

The author declared no conflict of interest.

Author details

Sumitra Debnath
College of Veterinary Science, Assam Agricultural University, Khanapara, Guwahati, India

*Address all correspondence to: sumitradebnath99@gmail.com

IntechOpen

References

[1] Dadpour B, Tajoddini S, Rjabi M, Afshari R. Mushroom poisoning in the northeast of Iran; a retrospective 6-year epidemiologic study. Emergency. 2017;**5**(1):e23

[2] Chauhan P, Singh B, Gupta S, Jeena Kumar N, Kumar D. Mushroom Diversity and their Biochemical Composition. London: Elite Publishing House; 2025

[3] Ahlawat OP, Tewari RP. Cultivation Technology of Paddy Straw Mushroom. HP: ICAR-DMR; 2007

[4] Cooke MC. Handbook of British Fungi. Vol. 1. London: Macmillan and Co; 1871. p. 138

[5] Ragul M. Exploration of antimicrobial potentials of fungal chitosan and secondary metabolites against soil borne plant pathogens [dissertation]. Coimbatore: Tamil Nadu Agricultural University; 2013

[6] Wieland T, Faulstich H. Amatoxins, phallotoxins, phallolysin, and antamanide: The biologically active components of poisonous amanita mushrooms. CRC Critical Reviews in Biochemistry. 1978;**5**:185-260

[7] Rohrmoser M, Kirchmair M, Feifel E, Valli A, Corradini R, Pohanka E, et al. Orella- nine poisoning: Rapid detection of the fun-gal toxin in renal biopsy material. Journal of Toxicology—Clinical Toxicology. 1997;**35**(1):63-66

[8] Letschert K, Faulstich H, Keller D, Keppler D. Molecular characterization and inhibition of amanitin uptake into human hepatocytes. Toxicological Sciences. 2016;**91**:140-149

[9] Zheleva A. Phenoxyl radicals formation might contribute to severe toxicity of mushroom toxin alpha-amanitin -an electron paramagnetic resonance study. TJS. 2013;**11**(1):33-38

[10] Bonnet X, Shine R, Lourdais O. Taxonomic chauvinism. Trends in Ecology & Evolution. 2002;**17**(1):861-864

[11] Jander S (Bischoff J. 2000), Treatment of *Amanita phalloides* poisoning: I. Retrospective evaluation of plasmapheresis in 21 patients. Therapeutic Apheresis; 4: 303-307

[12] Garcia J, Costa VM, Costa AE, Andrade S, Carneiro AC, Conceicao F, 2015. et al. Co-ingestion of amatoxins and isoxazoles-containing mushrooms and successful treatment: A case report. Toxicon; 103: 55-59.

[13] Escudié et al. *Amanita phalloides* poisoning: Reassessment of prognostic factors indications for emergency liver transplantation. Toxicon. 1999;**46**:466-473

[14] Singer R. Mushroom and Truffles: Botany, Cultivation and Utilization. London: Leonard Hill; 1961

[15] Chang ST. A cytological study of spore germination of Volvariella volvacea. Botanical Magazine. 1969;**82**:102109

[16] Eren SH, Demirel Y, Uğurlu S, Korkmaz I, Aktaş C, Guven FM. Mushroompoisoning: Retrospective analysis of 294 cases. Clinics (São Paulo, Brazil). 2010;**1**(65):491-496

[17] Michelot D, Melendez-Howel LM. *Amanita muscaria*: Chemistry, biology, toxicology, and ethnomycology. Mycological Research. 2003;**107**:131-146

[18] Berger KJ, Guss DA. Mycotoxins revisited: Part II. The Journal of Emergency Medicine. 2005;**28**:175-183

[19] Vendramin A, Brvar M. *Amanita muscaria* and amanita pantherina poisoning: Two syndromes. Toxicon. 2014;**90**:269-272

[20] Satora L, Pach D, Ciszowski K, Winnik L. Panther cap *Amanita pantherine* poisoning case report and review. Toxicon. 2006;**47**:605-607

Chapter 5

Assaults with Highly Toxic Substances in Public Spaces: Preparedness in Lessons Learnt from Precedent Cases

Martin Socher, Katrin Romanek, Thomas Zilker,
Hermann Fromme and Manfred Wildner

Abstract

The use of chemical substances in terrorist scenarios is to be feared everywhere. Especially after the events that have attracted attention in recent years such as the incident of a Sarin assault on Tokyo subway on March 20th 1995. In addition, the attacks with Novichok on the former Russian double agent Sergei Skripal in Salisbury, March 4th 2018, as well as on the prominent Russian opposition leader Alexei Navalny during a flight from Tomsk to Moscow on August 20th 2020 affected not only paramedics but also civilians in public areas. In order to collaterally protect civilian populations in the event of an emergency, the poisoning pattern (toxidrome) must be recognized as quickly and reliably as possible. Training on the relevant agents is needed and provision of necessary rescue equipment (antidotes) in prepared facilities is urgently required. In the event of a terrorist-motivated chemical attack, physicians from the Public Health Service (PHS) will foreseeably play a key role in communicating with decision-makers and the public as part of a competency network. As part of their preparation, the participants in the Bavarian Public Health training course are instructed in clinical symptomatology, toxicodynamics and therapy in the event of exposition to the most menacing, highly toxic chemical substances like organophosphorus (OP) compounds or vesicants such as Sulfur Mustard.

Keywords: chemical substances, terrorism, antidotes, Public Health Service, poison center

1. Introduction

The recent use of Sarin in Syria [1], the assassination of Kim Jong-Nam with VX in Malaysia [2] and the attack on Sergei Skripal with Novichok [3] underscore the persistent threat posed by organophosphorus (OP)-based nerve agents [4]. Since the 1930s, when Gerhard Schrader first discovered highly toxic OP compounds during

IntechOpen

pesticide research, there has been an ongoing effort to improve medical countermeasures and methods for early diagnosis of nerve agent poisoning. Upon exposure to an OP nerve agent (OPNA), the critical enzyme acetylcholinesterase (AChE) becomes inhibited through covalent binding of the agent to the active site serine. This inhibition results in the accumulation of the neurotransmitter acetylcholine at cholinergic synapses, followed by a cholinergic crisis owing to the overstimulation of cholinergic receptors, resulting in muscarinic and nicotinic signs. Among the muscarinic ones are salivation, lacrimation, urination, diarrhea, gastrointestinal distress and emesis; among the nicotinic ones are a broad spectrum of striated muscle dysfunction, including muscle weakness, fasciculations, with finally flaccid paralysis because of permanent depolarization. Central nervous system (CNS) manifestations enfold the impairment of respiratory drive, the loss of consciousness and seizures. Inhibited AChE may reactivate spontaneously, be deliberately reactivated by the administration of an oxime or undergo an aging reaction by losing an alkyl group—thus being permanently inactivated. Immediate treatment with a muscarinic receptor antagonist and an oxime is the current strategy to improve the survival of poisoned patients. However, the therapeutic effectiveness of currently licensed oximes is limited, e.g., by their insufficiency in reactivating AChE inhibited by certain nerve agents (e.g., Tabun), the inability of oximes to cross the blood-brain barrier and an aged form of AChE that cannot be reactivated [5, 6]. A meaningful part of the above-mentioned preparedness would be to prepare also physicians from PHS in terms of content for the case of an assault with highly toxic chemical substances. Although they would not be part of the responsible rescue team there is likelihood for them to be questioned as experts on the risk of the exposed population from mayors or district administrators. For such a case of emergency, a bioterrorist assault for example, it is to fear that major stress for the clinical supply system would arise from worried well who could multiply the number of truly injured people. This was already demonstrated by the precedent assault with Sarin on the Tokyo subway on March 20th 1995 [7]. For a necessary development of information materials and behavioral codes for the public during and after an assault with chemical substances, the PHS may account for the preservation of civil society and relief of clinical care from worried well [8]. Subsequently, there is some introductive information compiled on known substances like nerve agents, vesicants or opioids and experiences from incidents in recent years.

2. Nerve agents

One of the most feared chemical substance groups, nerve agents, blocks the organisms' cholinesterases, specifically the serums' pseudocholinesterase (butyrylcholinesterase (BChE)) whose activity is crucial for assessing the course of intoxication. It behaves like the neuronal cholinesterase, whose inhibition determines the patient's clinical picture. After elimination of the nerve agent's "leaving group" (X-group) (**Figure 1**), which determines the speed of the effects' onset, acetylcholinesterase (AChE) will be inhibited by phosphorylation of a specific serine residue in the enzyme's esteratic center. This reaction occurs more or less quickly after exposure to nerve agents. The loss of AChE function causes the complete peripheral, autonomic and central nervous systems to be permanently overstimulated, leading to a cholinergic crisis. Understanding the further biochemical reaction in nerve agent poisoning is crucial for assessing therapeutic options. The loss of alkyl residues (R1, R2) (**Figure 1**) from the nerve agent-cholinesterase complex is called "aging" and results

R1

|

R2 – P = O

|

X

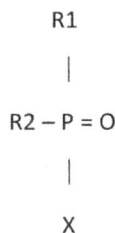

Figure 1.
Structural formula by Schrader.

in an irreversible, non-influenceable inhibition of AChE. Such a condition occurs within minutes of exposure to Soman (GD) (the half-life of Soman-AChE-complex is about 2 minutes), whereas it takes considerably longer after exposure to Sarin (GB) (half-life of 3 hours) and VX (half-life of 30 hours).

The organophosphorus substances were first synthesized by the politically aligned German dye industry, originally in search of insecticides before and during World War II. Gerhard Schrader synthesized Tabun (GA) in 1936 and Sarin (GB) in 1938, while Richard Kuhn, Nobel laureate in Chemistry in 1938, developed Soman (GD) in 1943. Further developments followed in England by the group surrounding British chemist Ghosh with VX in 1949. Its production rights were transferred to the US. The development of additional isomers followed in Russia (Russian VX (RVX)) and China (Chinese VX (CVX)). VX and its analogs belong to the so-called V (venomous) substances, which are phosphorylated thiocholine compounds without electron-donating groups, making them resistant to hydrolysis. This characteristic, combined with their very low volatility, ensures that these substances can be absorbed through unprotected skin into the bloodstream. Novichok was developed in the former USSR's "FOLIANT" project in the 1970s as a third-generation nerve agent with an organo-phosphorus structure, leading to at least four so-called A-agents (Substance-33, A230, A232, A234), with undetermined structures that could potentially be used in binary systems (Novichok-#, -5, -7), which are likely 5–10 times more effective than VX. The lethal dose 50% (LD50) of Novichok substances shall come up with 0.22 µg/kg that of 2-(dimethylamino)ethyl N,N-dimethylphosphoramidofluoridate (VG), a further new nerve agent of fourth generation [9]. Regarding therapeutic approaches, there are no differences from other organophosphorus compounds. After decontaminating the skin, the administration of anticholinergics Atropine, anticonvulsants (Diazepam) and oximes is indicated. However, the use of oximes would have a limited nucleophilic effect due to the A-agent already being complexed with AChE. Sarin and Soman are predominantly volatile substances, so their incorporation is expected mainly through inhalation. Cyclosarin (GF) and Tabun have more persistent properties, so their uptake can also occur through the skin. VX, in contrast, primarily develops its effects through skin contact.

2.1 Nerve agents' effects

In the early phase or in cases of minor poisoning, sympathetic symptoms are present due to preganglionic cholinergic transmission, with tachycardia and hyper-tension being predominant. As the parasympathetic response predominates, the typical symptoms of organophosphorus poisoning emerge, including hypersecretion of bronchial glands, bronchial muscle contractions, profuse sweating, salivation and tearing due to muscarinic overstimulation of exocrine glands. In the somatomotor system, nicotinic overstimulation causes symptoms such as eyelid tremors, contractions of facial muscles and muscle fibers, eventually leading to flaccid paralysis due to continuous depolarization. In the central nervous system (CNS), a cholinergic crisis causes dizziness, restlessness, speech disorders, loss of motor coordination, seizures and coma via muscarinic and nicotinic pathways. Fatality can result from central respiratory failure and pulmonary edema, which in severe cases may be accompanied by cardiovascular collapse.

Given this, it is essential to involve physicians from Public Health Service (PHS) during a terrorist chemical assault. While they may not directly care for casualties, they can be consulted by authorities and the press as experts on existing threats to the general population. In emergencies, such as the suspected bioterrorist attacks like those during New York City's 9/11 attacks and its extension to Afghanistan [8], there is concern that the number of casualties could increase due to the "worried well," who might misinterpret the danger and add pressure to clinical systems, as seen in the 1995 Tokyo Sarin attack. To effectively handle such situations, including public information and rules of conduct, PHS can help maintain a functioning civil society at the regional level, manage the concerns of the worried well and ensure access to specialized staff for diagnosis and poison information, thus preventing unnecessary visits to clinical centers [6].

The "worried well" often overestimate their exposure to poison, influenced by media coverage of actual victims, which they cannot differentiate due to fear, lack of experience and knowledge. Information materials should be distributed in advance to guide people on how to act in situations where they perceive potential danger [8].

The most important measures in an emergency are ensuring that emergency services are trained to recognize the signs and symptoms of life-threatening events in which poisoning is not only possible but highly likely due to the circumstances. Securing the availability of crucial supplies (antidotes, decontamination materials, personal protective equipment (PPE)), and the transfer of affected individuals to more specialized institutions, if necessary is vital. It is also important to secure specimens from affected patients for poison detection and forensic examination. On-site diagnostic capabilities, such as detecting acetylcholinesterase (AChE) activity or spot contamination, should be available, and action teams should be equipped with self-protection gear.

2.2 Experiences of assaults with nerve agents

Lessons to be learnt in the management of nerve agents arose from the Japanese Sarin attacks carried out by Aum Shinrikyo on June 27th 1994 when the politically motivated cult released about 20–30 kg of Sarin through the window of a converted delivery truck and spread the substance over a residential area in Matsumoto to poison three district court judges, thus trying to preempt an anticipated unfavorable ruling.

Some 600 people were exposed, 253 sought medical attention at outpatient clinics. The majority suffered from decreased visual acuity and miosis (n = 57). There were 58 patients admitted to hospitals and all recovered. Seven casualties living close to the release of the chemical died before getting to the hospital and the judges, who were the primary targets, survived. The death toll from the assault would probably have been higher if the release of the Sarin had been more efficient.

On March 20th 1995, members of the same sect released an estimated 4.5 L of dissolved Sarin on five central line subway trains in Tokyo during the morning rush hour. First emergency calls reached the fire department within 20 minutes from 15 different stations. Authorities at first did not understand that the emergency had a single cause. Arriving at the scene, rescue teams found commuters stumbling about with impaired vision, struggling to breathe. Casualties littered the subway station exits, some foaming at the mouth, some vomiting and others convulsing. Inside subway stations and near the exits, rescue teams began to triage victims and offer medical assistance, although they administered no drugs and did not intubate serious cases at the scene. Nor did they decontaminate the victims, but took the most seriously affected patients to hospital.

Over 5000 "casualties" sought medical attention, 984 persons were moderately and 54 persons severely poisoned, 12 died [7].

Making a correct diagnosis was challenging due to discordant vegetative signs (tachycardia on one hand but miosis on the other hand) in the course of early or mild intoxication. False diagnosis occurred based on suspicion (e.g., Acetonitrile) in an unclear and confusing situation, complete with an obvious lack of necessary information and means for detection.

The Sarin assault in Tokyo is the most well-documented case of mass intoxication. Leading symptoms consisted of miosis (99%) with a severe headache (83%), dyspnea (70%) and nausea (67%). Further emesis, weakness, fasciculations and obtundation were visible. Some classic muscarinic signs like sweating, salivation and lacrimation were astonishingly less observed. The miosis was caused by local contamination of the eye.

In the cases of Navalny and Skripal, two further poisoning incidents with nerve agents (see further down), unconsciousness occurred soon after a short phase of nausea. While the suppression of cholinesterase by volatile nerve agents endures for only a short time (1 day), it lasts for several days in fluid and solid substances like VX and Novichok. With Soman and Tabun, the application of an oxime remains ineffective, whereas with Sarin, VX and also Novichok an early application might be helpful. In Navalny's case, it occurred too late [5, 10].

In Tokyo, most affected individuals were taken to hospital without prior on-site decontamination, which should have been done urgently to avoid exposing hospital staff to secondary toxin exposure. The same problem emerged due to the non-availability of personal protective equipment (PPE) in hospitals, and therefore adequate decontamination procedures could not be conducted there. Thus, 23% of 472 staff members in St. Luke's Hospital complained of acute symptoms of secondary toxin exposure but none of them got any treatment. Besides that, a lack of essential antidotes (Atropine, Oximes) was registered at the scene [7].

2.3 Experiences from life-threatening, politically motivated incidents with nerve agents

On February 13th 2017, two women both rubbed the face of Kim Jong-Nam, half-brother of the North Korean dictator, at Kuala Lumpur International Airport, Malaysia for 7 seconds with four low-toxic starting substances that reacted to VX on his eyes and skin. This led to his death within 20 minutes. Although the two assassins had not worn gloves, they were little affected by the poison. The chemical analysis by the Malaysian government indicated that Kim indeed was killed by VX.

VX was likely synthesized from several precursor compounds applied sequentially by the two women involved in the attack. The binary VX system developed by the U.S. Army consists of two components: QL (isopropyl aminoethylmethyl phosphonite) and rhombic sulfur. However, Malaysian police reported that QL was not detected on either of the women's hands or on Kim Jong-Nam himself.

A key observation was that the chemical compounds identified from the three individuals—the two attackers and the victim—were all different, which strongly suggests the use of a binary nerve agent system. This is particularly compelling, given the stark differences between the substances found on each woman. If preformed VX had been used instead of a binary system, one would expect the same compound to be present on both women.

On the Indonesian woman's T-shirt, ethyl methylphosphonic acid was detected. Meanwhile, samples from the Vietnamese woman's T-shirt and fingernails contained 2-(diisopropylamino)ethyl chloride, 2-(diisopropylamino)ethanethiol and bis(2-diisopropylaminoethyl) disulfide. These findings support the hypothesis that VX was formed directly on Kim's face after the second woman applied the final component with her palm.

Kim's complaint of eye pain shortly after the attack suggests that the nerve agent entered his body through ocular tissues, causing both immediate irritation and rapid systemic absorption. This could explain his death within 20 minutes of exposure. It is likely that a lethal dose of VX was absorbed through the mucous membranes of his eyes [2, 11, 12].

On March 4th 2018, Sergei Skripal, a former Russian double agent, and his daughter, were poisoned with Novichok (Engl. "newcomer") in Salisbury by touching a primed door handle. They both collapsed on a bench close to the restaurant where they had eaten. The cause was not immediately obvious but it was recognized rapidly that they had been exposed to some toxic substance. A policeman was also exposed to what appeared to be the same substance while helping the Skripals. He was initially discharged from the hospital, but his condition deteriorated at home and he was readmitted there. With treatment, the three patients recovered, the Skripals were however discharged at least 2 weeks later because of their stronger exposition. Although 46 members of the public presented themselves at the hospital expressing concern and a further 131 people had been identified who could potentially have come into contact with the nerve agent, the Consultant in Emergency Medicine at the Salisbury NHS hospital stated that nevertheless no one other than the known three patients had needed treatment. On March 7th 2018, it was announced by the then Prime Minister (PM) that the Skripals had been exposed to a "nerve agent" and on March 12th that this was a Novichok nerve agent. This finding by the Defense Science and Technology Laboratory (DSTL), Porton Down was confirmed independently by the Organisation for the Prohibition of Chemical Weapons (OPCW), The Hague, on collected environmental samples. A woman, who found the used transport vessel in nearby Amesbury some months later, mistook its content and used it as a perfume, which caused her death from severe intoxication 8 days later [3].

On August 20th 2020, 44-year-old Alexei Navalny, a well-known Russian opposition activist, who was previously healthy suddenly became confused and began to sweat heavily on a domestic flight within Russia approximately 10 minutes after departure; he vomited, collapsed and lost consciousness. After an emergency landing, the man was admitted to a local hospital in Omsk, Siberia, approximately 2 hours after symptom onset. According to the discharge report, the patient presented comatose with hypersalivation and increased diaphoresis and was diagnosed with respiratory failure, myoclonic status, disturbed carbohydrate metabolism, electrolyte disorders and metabolic encephalopathy. Therapeutic measures included intubation, mechanical ventilation and unspecified drugs for symptom control and neuroprotection. On August 22nd 2020, the patient was transferred by German air ambulance to the Charité University Hospital in Berlin at the request of his family. Severe poisoning with a cholinesterase inhibitor was subsequently diagnosed. Two weeks later, the German Government announced that the Institute of Pharmacology and Toxicology of the German Armed Forces in Munich, designated by the Organization for the Prohibition of Chemical Weapons (OPCW), had identified an organophosphorus nerve agent from the Novichok group in blood samples collected immediately after the patient's admission to Charité, a finding that was subsequently confirmed by the OPCW [10].

Mr. Navalny, who returned to Russia pretty directly after his discharge from the university hospital in Berlin, was immediately arrested at the airport because of alleged treason and finally died on January 16th 2024 in a prison in Siberia's northern polar circle from unknown reasons.

2.4 Nerve agents' poisoning effects and treatment

Nerve agents block the cholinesterases of all organisms by phosphorylation and thereby lead to a cholinergic overstimulation of the vegetative nervous system, the so-called cholinergic crisis. The inhibition of the neuronal cholinesterase determines the clinical picture of exposed patients, which merges into a reactivation-refractory, virtually irreversible inhibition depending on differences in time latency of the aging of poison-enzyme-complexes. This may lead to pre- and postganglionic caused discordant vegetative signs (e.g., miosis versus sympathicotonic vital parameters), which can cause clinical confusion among the physicians responsible for the first view on the case. Point-of-care devices for detection of erythrocyte acetylcholinesterase (EryAChE) are generally available and can ease diagnostic procedures considerably. They help to confirm a clinical suspicion of intoxication with nerve agents so that an adequate therapy can be initiated within minutes. Therefore, rescue teams should have them at hand. Initially, Atropine is able to treat and secure respiration and circulation by blocking muscarinic acetylcholine receptors. Starting with 2 mg, the dose can be doubled depending on patient's response, although 10 mg already constitutes a fairly high dose above which overdosing should be avoided. The dose for affected children has to be adapted critically, according to their ages or, if known, weight (0.02–0.1 mg/kg).

The control of cerebral seizures by an appropriate dose of Atropine is not possible. For this purpose, Diazepam 10–20 mg should be administered intravenously and repeated as necessary, usually once or twice, maximum three times per day under stationary conditions only.

Atropine has no influence on the functional paralysis of the respiratory muscles caused by nicotinic acetylcholine receptors, which is why attempts should be made to restore the neuromuscular transmission by application of an acetylcholinesterase reactivator. This approach at all synapses, also the parasympathetic ones, should help to save a large amount of Atropine doses. If this approach is effective it is also highly efficient, though subject to substance-specific limitations. As, for example, the Soman-AChE-complex ages within minutes and reactivation is no longer achievable after a short time. In addition, the currently known and available oximes, Obidoxime and the less effective Pralidoxime, show no broadband effect on all relevant organophosphorus substances and pesticides acting in the same manner. A causal therapy is therefore not available for all substances. In the case of mass poisoning with Sarin/VX however, a reactivation could still be possible within hours. In cases with longer persisting substances with a prolonged cholinergic crisis, a continual atropinization (clinical criteria: free respiratory sounds on auscultation, heart rate > 80 beats/min, pupils>pinpoint, dry axilla skin, blood pressure > 80 mmHg) of exposed people can be necessary. In the event of an emergency, sufficient amounts of antidotes for several hundred victims must be held available in depots. Their use on severely poisoned persons in the field is made more difficult for the emergency services due to their obligation to wear protective suits. Recommendations in this regard are therefore discussed in a controversial manner but seem possible to implement with repeated training of the personal while wearing protective equipment. This should be held available at all disposable rescue centers. If reactivation fails, severely affected patients have to be ventilated mechanically until spontaneous respiration sufficiently recovers. An orientation of approximately 20% of normal butyrylcholinesterase (BChE) activity as reference for spontaneous recovery is only a rough indicator. Nevertheless, an inclining BChE activity shows a decreasing inhibition. The preferred surrogate parameter for neuromuscular transmission is EryAChE, which corresponds to neuronal AChE but its analysis is not readily available. This should be improved urgently for the case of an emergency. Decontamination by disrobing should be initiated before a transfer or at least before admission to hospital followed by showering in special decontamination units. Hospitals should also be prepared to proceed in the same manner with patients who self-present because adequate protection for their staff and facilities is of the highest importance [13].

2.5 Management of antidotal treatment in severe nerve agent intoxication

Atropine binds competitively to all muscarinic receptors without activating them. Therefore, it is the optimal means for replacing acetylcholine from these receptors and eliminating parts of the toxic effect. The nicotinic effects however stay unaffected, which means that the central nervous, ganglionic and muscular nicotinic effects remain after Atropine administration. Furthermore, patients can exhibit severe nicotine poisoning and therefore remain in need of ventilation and sedation. The most important life-saving effects of Atropine are the relief of bronchial spasms, bronchorrhea and bradycardia, raising the threshold for cerebral seizures and a favorable effect on the circulation. It should be dosed at 2 mg intravenously and its dose doubled every 5 minutes dependent on the patient's clinical response. In mass poisoning, the dose can only be given intramuscularly. The usual maintenance dose is 2 mg per hour. A sign that is easy to monitor is the pupil size, which is practical at the beginning of the poisoning when the pupil should only be of an average size. In the further course of treatment, pupil size is influenced by different sedatives and becomes less reliable for the assessment of the correct Atropine dose. More important than pupil size are, of course, the cardiovascular parameters that serve as a control for the Atropine dosage. A heart rate of 80–100 beats/min should be aimed for. However, this parameter becomes less valuable when, as it is very often the case, emerging pneumonia with the development of fever and tachycardia occurs. In this situation, the assessment of bronchorrhea is suitable for dosage control: there should be no more spasticity and crepitation on auscultation and little or no secretions. This parameter, too, becomes unreliable in the long term due to the pneumonia, which itself leads to secretions and crepitations. Beyond that, the assessment of diaphoresis, salivation and bowel sounds can be used. Again, bowel sounds are not very consistent as they appear to respond to lower doses of Atropine than the other parameters. The remaining signs are considered to be diaphoresis and salivation. The cessation of the former can best be examined under the axilla, the latter by suction of the salvia in the mouth. Besides finding the optimal dosage, there is a further problem with atropinization. The gastrointestinal tract reacts most sensitively to Atropine, which can induce constipation on a relatively low dose of it. It also seems that adaption phenomena can arise, leading to a kind of "rebound" when stopping the Atropine therapy: This means that clear cholinergic signs can occur, even though no poisoning persists. Such a phase can be tolerated in a relaxed manner if the butyrylcholinesterase (BChE) or erythrocyte AChE (EryAChE) has already been increased [13].

Unfortunately, oxime antidotes do not act equally in all poisonings with phosphororganic toxins. In rapidly aging substances like Soman and dimethyl organophosphates, they work only when used very early after exposition. After sometime, reactivation is no longer possible due to the loss of the alkyl chains from their benzene rings. For this case, there are autoinjectors available, containing Atropine and an oxime, to improve the prognosis of exposed and symptomatic victims. In contrast, reactivation is successful with diethyl-organophosphates and several nerve agents, which split only slowly with aging half-lives of about 3 hours (Sarin) and some 36–40 hours (VX, diethyl-organophosphorus compounds). As the causative phosphororganic substance is usually unknown at the beginning of the poisoning, Obidoxime 250 mg should always be administered as a bolus as early as possible and be continued as an infusion at 30 mg/h or 750 mg/day. The first step of the oxime-induced reactivation is the additional binding of the oxime via a nitrogen atom to the phosphorylated acetylcholinesterase (AChE). This first step is dependent on the concentration of the reactivator and follows a dose-effect relationship. The second step describes the original reactivation. The oxime thereby escapes from the enzyme together with the phosphoryl residue of the toxin, a phosphoryloxime is formed and the serine residue of the AChE is released. This second step always takes place at the same rate, independent of the concentration of the oxime. Increasing the oxime dose therefore remains ineffective. A continuous increase in the dose should therefore be avoided but a concentration of 10–20 µmol/L Obidoxime in serum should be maintained long enough for maximal efficacy. Thereby, the effectiveness of oximes in severe poisonings with phosphororganic compounds is limited. In such cases, the inactivation of AChE by organophosphorus compounds may be faster than the reactivation by the oxime. Because this cannot be predicted in individual cases, a standardized procedure should initially be applied in all poisonings [13, 14].

To control the seizures triggered by nerve agents, benzodiazepines are effective anticonvulsants. Diazepam 10–20 mg should be administered intravenously and repeated as necessary under medical supervision and readiness for intubation. An alternative is Midazolam 10 mg, then a repeated dose of 10 mg after 10 minutes if required, but it offers no advantages over Diazepam [7].

3. Vesicants (blister agents)

The most important blister agent is Sulfur Mustard, a simple chemical substance called dichlorodiethyl sulfide. Various other names are S-Lost after the names of the two German chemists Lommel and Steinkopf who first proposed its suitability for widespread use as chemical warfare agent, and Yperit named after Ypern, the Belgian site of its first use during World War I on July 12th 1917. Under normal environmental conditions, sulfur mustard is a fluid, which is why it has to be deployed as an aerosol to become maximally bioavailable, though it is questionable if this advanced technology was conceivable in Gulf War I or even World War I. Mustard gas is irritating to the eyes, skin and bronchial mucous membranes, manifesting itself, dependent on the concentration of poison, with a time latency of some hours. Initially, it reacts highly sensitively on the conjunctiva with lacrimation and light sensitivity, irritation, eye-lid spasms and pyogenic conjunctivitis. The skin shows rubor and edema with severe pruritus, which after prolonged or severe exposure transitions into painful, fluid-filled vesicles that are fully developed after 12–24 hours and which can lead to deep pyogenic ulcers. The susceptibility of the skin increases with the density of the sweating and sebaceous glands and typically shows affected areas in juxtaposition with discoloration. Initial respiratory symptoms are catarrhal disturbances, dry throat, hoarseness and aphonia, followed by purulent bronchitis and bronchopneumonia. They can also be accompanied by the formation of pseudomembranes and obstruction of the airways. Immunosuppression caused by hematopoietic failure in the bone marrow can contribute to the death of patients. Due to the lack of a specific antidote, the first step in the treatment chain consists of a careful decontamination of the affected persons using appropriate self-protection measures by the rescue team (protective suit, special gloves, boots, breathing mask). Skin lesions caused by Sulfur Mustard should be treated as burns that are complicated by a reduced wound healing. Ideally, the body surface should be dabbed with a paste containing hypochlorite early on, eyes must be flushed with water or 2% sodium bicarbonate liquid and the systemic effect can be avoided by infusion of sodium thiosulfate liquid, but this is only effective within 20 minutes of exposure. Clearing the bronchial system by tracheotomy and bronchoscopic debridement can save the victim from suffocation. Secondary infections have to be treated by antibiotics locally and systemically, according to the microbial sensitivity testing [5, 13, 15–17].

3.1 Experiences in poisoning with vesicants

The devastating effect of Sulfur Mustard has been known in Europe since World War I. Since then, severely wounded Iranians from the First Gulf War have also been treated in Germany and other parts of Europe. There were only a few fatal poisonings—possibly a selection bias in patients deemed fit enough to be transferred to Europe—but severe and permanent skin and tracheal disorders were observed. In these cases, enough time was available to provide medication, decontamination, repeated wound dressings and to take general care of those affected, if necessary over several weeks in hospital. However, in the case of a more severe involvement of the lungs, the prognosis could have been worse. The effective management of multiple assaults can obviously be very critical and may also lead to a burden of a country's health system in the long term [16, 17].

In mass poisoning, there will be an enormous workload on the hospitals that could interfere with the care of other patients. Sequelae on the lungs and eyes were common with obstructive pulmonary disease and secondary blindness.

4. Opioids

After the occupation of a musical theater in Moscow by Chechen terrorists on October 26th 2002 and the ensuing hostage rescue attempt by Russian authorities, the undisclosed use of inhalative Carfentanil and Remifentanil via the ventilation system of the building led to the death of 127 (16%) of the 800 hostages in the theater and of at least 33 hostage-takers. All suffered from an undetected opioid intoxication, although classical signs (unconsciousness, respiratory depression, pinpoint pupils) were present. The Russian government had not revealed the used composition of the inserted aerosol, in public it was even presumed the application of highly toxic warfare compounds like Sarin, VX or BZ. After laboratory-analyzed findings of clothes and blood samples of two British survivors and a urine sample of a third survivor with Russian name by the DSTL, Porton Down, UK as well as urine samples of two other patients, evacuated by the German air ambulance to the Department of Clinical Toxicology of the Technical University of Munich (TU Munich), in which the Centers for Disease Control and Prevention (CDC), Atlanta, USA could verify Norcarfentanil and Remifentanil metabolites, there is evidence to suggest that the used aerosol in the theater at Moscow had consisted of a mixture of Carfentanil and Remifentanil. A fast loss of consciousness after inhalation of the aerosol and analgesia after awakening, as reported exemplarily by the first two mentioned patients, coincides with the effect of these fentanyl derivatives. These opioids are clinically used as injection narcotics—Carfentanil thereby possesses a 10,000-fold effectiveness of Morphine and is accredited only for use in animals— leading to anesthesia, analgesia and undesirable depression of breathing. Both substances have an only narrow therapeutic margin and Carfentanil could have been mixed with the smaller and shorter-acting Remifentanil to decrease the number of casualties that would have been resulted by a sole use of the former. The use of the indicated antidote Naloxon in this case could probably have saved a large number of lives if the nature of the used substances had been known or the clinical conditions of the casualties had been better recognized. Naloxon is a pure antagonist to all opioid receptors studied to date and is therefore able to antagonize all the effects of Morphine and further agonistic-acting substances [18]. The lives of the surviving 650 hostages were probably saved by the intervention of the Russian state as the terrorists were planning to explode the building.

5. Management of warfare agent attacks

Early decontamination is essential and should begin with the removal of the patient's clothing and thorough washing of the skin, while ensuring the responder is properly protected with specialized gear—such as butyl rubber gloves, gas masks, vinyl footwear and protective overgarments. Stabilization of vital functions and prompt evacuation from the hazardous area must also be prioritized. In cases involving nerve agents or vesicants, immediate skin decontamination is especially critical. It is only effective against vesicants when performed without delay and is vital for preventing skin absorption and systemic toxicity—particularly with low-volatility nerve agents like VX.

The first and most crucial step is the rapid removal of contaminated clothing. The effectiveness of decontamination diminishes over time, as chemical agents may permeate clothing, increasing the risk of cutaneous absorption under occlusive conditions. Skin decontamination methods fall into two categories: dry and wet. Dry decontamination involves the use of adsorbent powders such as fuller's earth, which remove liquid agents from the skin. However, care must be taken to prevent the generation of contaminated dust, which could pose an inhalation hazard.

Wet decontamination entails the use of large volumes of plain water, sometimes combined with surfactants such as soap or detergents to enhance solubility and removal of oily substances like VX.

The U.S. Food and Drug Administration (FDA) has endorsed the integration of decontamination and detoxification into a single step. Reactive skin decontamination lotion (RSDL), which contains 2,3-butanedione monoxime, polyethylene glycol and solvents, is specifically formulated to aid in the desorption of nerve agents from the skin and their subsequent breakdown via nucleophilic reaction. RSDL has demonstrated superior efficacy in treating percutaneous VX exposure compared to conventional decontamination agents such as fuller's earth. Overall, the first step in the effective treatment of nerve agent or vesicant poisoning must incorporate advanced and rapid decontamination and detoxification strategies [1, 19].

In cases where oral exposure is suspected in an unconscious patient, the administration of 50 g of medical charcoal via gastric tube should be considered, while ensuring that aspiration is avoided. Laxatives are generally unnecessary, as patients typically present with diarrhea [13].

5.1 Triage in mass casualty incidents involving toxic chemicals

In the aftermath of a chemical attack involving highly toxic substances and multiple casualties, establishing a triage protocol is essential. Given the likelihood of resource constraints, patients must be prioritized based on medical urgency:

- *First priority*: Patients in critical condition who can be stabilized if intensive care unit (ICU) resources are available.

- *Second priority*: Patients requiring immediate life-saving interventions within the next hour.

- *Third priority*: Patients with moderate injuries who can safely await delayed treatment or transport.

- *Fourth priority*: Patients in terminal condition who are unlikely to survive, even with antidote administration. These individuals should receive palliative care.

- *Fifth priority*: Patients at risk of delayed respiratory distress due to inhalation of pulmonary agents (choking agents). These individuals require observation for at least 24 hours following antidote administration.

5.2 Zoning and site management

At the scene, the incident commander must define the geographic extent of the affected zones. The *hot zone* (black area) represents the immediate contamination site and may extend up to 1 kilometer (km), depending on meteorological conditions, terrain and the volatility of the chemical agents involved. Surrounding this is the *warm zone* (gray area), where medical stabilization and decontamination procedures are performed to prevent secondary contamination. Beyond this lies the *cold zone* (white area), where the lead emergency physician coordinates patient triage and distribution to appropriate healthcare facilities [5].

6. Discussion

When preparing countermeasures against deliberate release of highly toxic compounds in public spaces, clinical toxicologists and poison centers, in particular, should play a complementary role, taking into account the responsibility of the designated emergency management authority and in cooperation with the PHS. In some emergency medical services, given the availability of a poison control center, there may also be toxicologically competent emergency physicians who can be called to the scene, if needed supported by a rescue helicopter to shorten transportation time and by the whole rescue system and whenever possible by the medical service of the armed forces. Diagnostic capacity, access to poison information by the worried well that place additional burdens on healthcare facilities and a sufficient supply of necessary antidotes and protective equipment for emergency responders and civilians on emergency management units are critical for a successful situation management.

In summary, these three elements—availability and access to specific diagnostic technology, therapeutic information for specialized staff in combination with an adequate stockpiling of antidotes and protective equipment—seem crucial for a preventive, public health-oriented preparedness for assaults with highly toxic substances in public spaces.

7. Materials and methods

A narrative review was compiled to present the actual level of knowledge in identification and handling of assaults with highly toxic chemical substances in public space. The experiences from incidents in recent years were given to colleagues in the field of public health at national congresses [5] who are supposed to have got a description of the theme's development as state of the art in presence, in how this understanding was reached and what may be expected from it prospectively.

The studied literature was collected by searching in www.pubmed.com using terms like GA, GB, GD, VX and references of found papers.

8. Conclusions

The recent use of nerve agents in military conflicts and assassination attempts has shown that the diagnosis and treatment of nerve agent exposure are an impending issue that has already made headlines at suitable occasions. The currently licensed oximes as antidotes have been in use for many decades, lacking the substantial improvement that still none of the available drugs can be used as a broad-spectrum oxime covering all relevant nerve agents and organophosphorus pesticides. Nevertheless, therapeutic gaps render further development crucial. The promising concept of a combination of different oximes with a complementary spectrum might be an interim solution to overcome current therapeutic limitations. A further corner-stone of nerve agent poisoning is the use of point-of-care diagnostics that render early diagnosis possible within 5 minutes by using a mobile ready-to-use kit to determine red blood cell AChE activity. Patients displaying inconclusive signs and symptoms might benefit from the therapeutic guidance these devices readily provide. Finally, the OP skin disclosure kit provides the opportunity to verify percutaneous exposure to low-volatility nerve agents, even before the first clinical signs occur [1, 19].

For the organization of concepts named under Discussion and their implementation, members of the PHS may assume a complementary role, for example as committed specialists in communal crisis teams and as communicators with health professionals, emergency services and the public. Confidence in reliable communication by actors of the state, an evidence-based approach and well-prepared, targeted purposeful measures, are essential, especially as comprehensive knowledge of the situation is still lacking. The present input wants to sensitize therefore and to deliver impulses for a review of existing preparedness. It does not claim a complete information about the complex issue, which probably underlies in parts also international confidentiality. Of special importance here is the additional coming into force of the "Chemical Weapons Convention (CWC) as Convention on the Prohibition of the Development, Production, Stockpiling and Use of Chemical Weapons and on their Destruction" in 1997, which was compiled by the member states of the United Nations (UN) in 1992 and since then the OPCW has been founded and instructed to control the convention committed of 193 states [20].

For further reasons, succeeding generations of colleagues, at least in the Bavarian PHS, are already being familiarized with a potential public risk posed by chemical substances possibly through terrorist learning from the experiences of recent years. This was conducted through lectures or, during the severe adult respiratory syndrome coronavirus II (SARS-CoV-II) pandemic, through suitable scripts containing the main information on clinical symptomatology, toxicodynamics and therapy in cases of exposition to the most menacing, highly toxic chemical substances such as organophosphorus compounds like Sarin or vesicants like Sulfur Mustard gas. From 2018 onward, these lessons have been given to participants of the Bavarian Public Health training course who have additionally come from further southern German federal states like Baden-Württemberg, Rhineland-Palatinate, Saarland, Saxony or Thuringia. As a shortcoming, it cannot, of course, be ruled out that the topic may not receive the desired attention as there is not enough lecture time given to the subject during the complete course for PHS training. This paper therefore aims to raise awareness on this topic in its entirety and provide an impulse for a review of existing preparatory work [5].

Conflict of interest

The authors declare no conflict of interests.

Abbreviations

AChE	acetylcholinesterase
BChE	butyrylcholinesterase
DSTL	Defence Science and Technology Laboratory
EryAChE	erythrocyte acetylcholinesterase
GA	Tabun
GB	Sarin
GD	Soman
NHS	National Health Service
OPCW	Organisation for the Prohibition of Chemical Weapons
PHS	Public Health Service
PPE	personal protective equipment

Assaults with Highly Toxic Substances in Public Spaces: Preparedness in Lessons Learnt...
DOI: http://dx.doi.org/10.5772/intechopen.1011887

QL	isopropyl aminoethylmethyl phosphonite
RVX	Russian VX
VG	2-(dimethylamino)ethyl N,N-dimethylphosphoramidofluoridate

Author details

Martin Socher[1,2]*, Katrin Romanek[2], Thomas Zilker[2], Hermann Fromme[3]
and Manfred Wildner[1,4]

1 Bavarian Authority of Health and Food Safety, Munich, Germany

2 Department of Clinical Toxicology, Medical Clinic II, Technical University Munich,
Munich, Germany

3 Institute and Outpatient Clinic for Occupational, Social and Environmental
Medicine Clinical Centre, Ludwig-Maximilians-University Munich, Munich,
Germany

4 Pettenkofer School of Public Health, Ludwig-Maximilians-University Munich,
Munich, Germany

*Address all correspondence to: martin.socher@lgl.bayern.de

IntechOpen

References

[1] Amend N, Niessen KV, Seeger T, Wille T, Worek F, Thiermann H. Diagnostics and treatment of nerve agent poisoning—Current status and future developments. Annals. New York Academy of Sciences. 2020;**1479**:13-28

[2] Nakagawa T, Tu AT. Murders with VX: Aum Shinrikyo in Japan and the assassination of Kim Jong-Nam in Malaysia. Forensic Toxicology. 2018;**36**:542-544

[3] Vale JA, Marrs TC, Maynard RL. Novichok: A murderous nerve agent attack in the UK. Clinical Toxicology. 2018;**56**(11):1093-1097

[4] OPCW. Practical Guide for Medical Management of Chemical Warfare Casualties, The Hague. 2024. Available from: https://www.opcw.org/resources/assistance-and-protection/practical-guide-medical-management-chemical-warfare-casualties

[5] Socher M, Zilker T, Fromme H, Wildner M. Preparation for attacks with highly toxic substances in public spaces. Gesundheitswesen. 2022;**84**:647-650. [in German]

[6] Socher M, Zilker T, Felgenhauer N, Fromme H, Wildner M. Terrorism with chemical substances. In: Wichmann, Fromme, editors. Handbook of Environmental Medicine. Vol. 71. Landsberg/Lech: Ecomed-Verlag; 2021. Erg.Lfg [in German]

[7] Vale JA. What lessons can we learn from the Japanese sarin attacks? Przegląd Lekarski. 2005;**62**:528-532

[8] Weinstein RS, Alibek K. Biological and Chemical Terrorism. Stuttgart, New York: Thieme Verlag; 2003

[9] Nepovimova E, Kuca K. Chemical warfare agent NOVICHOK—Mini-review of available data. Food and Chemical Toxicology. 2018;**121**:343-350

[10] Steindl D, Boehmerle W, Eckardt K-U, et al. Novichok nerve agent poisoning. Lancet. 2021;**397**:249-252

[11] Chai PR, Boyer EW, Al-Nahhas H, Erickson TB. Toxic chemical weapons of assassination and warfare: Nerve agents VX and sarin. Toxicology Communications. 2017;**1**(1):21-23

[12] Tu AT. The use of VX as a terrorist agent: Action by Aum Shinrikyo of Japan and the death of Kim Jong-Nam in Malaysia: Four case studies. Global Security: Health, Science and Policy. 2020;**5**(1):48-56

[13] Zilker T. Clinical Toxicology for Intensive Care Medicine: Toxins, Symptoms, Therapy, Analysis. 2. Auflage. Bremen: UNI-MED; 2023. [in German]

[14] Zilker T. Medical management of incidents with chemical warfare agents. Toxicology. 2005;**214**:221-231

[15] Wille T, Steinritz D, Worek F, Thiermann H. Poisoning from chemical warfare agents. Bundesgesundheitsblatt - Gesundheitsforschung - Gesundheitsschutz.2019;**62**(11):1370-1377. [in German]

[16] Willems JL. Clinical management of mustard gas casualties. Annales Medicinae Militaris Belgicae. 1989;**3**(Supplement):1-61

[17] Kehe K, Thiermann H, Balszuweit F, Eyer F, Steinritz D, Zilker T. Acute effects of sulfur

mustard injury—Munich experiences.
Toxicology. 2009;**263**(1):3-8

[18] Riches JR, Read RW, Black RM,
Cooper NJ, Timperley CM. Analysis of
clothing and urine from Moscow theatre
siege casualties reveals Carfentanil and
remifentanil use. Journal of Analytical
Toxicology. 2012;**36**:647-656

[19] Thiermann H, Worek F, Kehe K.
Limitations and challenges in
treatment of acute chemical warfare
agent poisoning. Chemico-Biological
Interactions. 2013;**206**:435-443

[20] Convention on the Prohibition of the
Development, Production, Stockpiling
and Use of Chemical Weapons and
on their Destruction. Available from:
https://www.opcw.org/sites/default/
files/documents/CWC/CWC_en.pdf
[Accessed: January 16, 2025]